C000023547

HAIR *POWER* – SKIN *REVOLUTION*

A collection of poems and personal essays
by black and mixed-race women

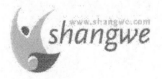

www.shangwe.com
shangwe

ALSO BY NICOLE MOORE

Sexual Attraction Revealed: A selection of creative expressions by black and mixed-race women – 2007 (editor)

Brown Eyes: A selection of creative expressions by black and mixed-race women – 2005 (editor)

HAIR *POWER*
SKIN *REVOLUTION*

A collection of poems and personal

essays by black and

mixed-race women

Edited by
Nicole Moore

Copyright © 2010 Nicole Moore

The moral right of the author has been asserted.

Apart from any fair dealing for the purposes of research or private study,
or criticism or review, as permitted under the Copyright, Designs and Patents
Act 1988, this publication may only be reproduced, stored or transmitted, in
any form or by any means, with the prior permission in writing of the
publishers, or in the case of reprographic reproduction in accordance with
the terms of licences issued by the Copyright Licensing Agency. Enquiries
concerning reproduction outside those terms should be sent to the publishers.

Matador
5 Weir Road
Kibworth
Leicester LE8 0LQ, UK
Tel: (+44) 116 2792299
Email: books@troubador.co.uk
Web: www.troubador.co.uk/matador

British Library Cataloguing in Publication Data.
A catalogue record for this book is available from the British Library.

ISBN 978 1848763 937

Typeset in 11pt Bookman by Troubador Publishing Ltd, Leicester, UK

LOTTERY FUNDED

Matador is an imprint of Troubador Publishing Ltd

Printed in Great Britain by the MPG Books Group, Bodmin and King's Lynn

For my granddaughter, Sophie

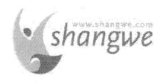

Shangwe is a female Swahili (East African) name
and means Celebration

CONTENTS

POEMS: SKIN   **167**

THE JOURNEY SO FAR: AN INTRODUCTION

My introduction to the world of literature came at a late age through an experience that stirred up all sorts of thoughts and emotions and I knew straight away that it was not just a world, but the world in which I wanted to live and work. It was the year 1995 when I studied black women's literature, which gave me the rare opportunity to delve, with others, into the worlds of African-Caribbean and Black British writers. I was able to deepen my understanding of issues affecting black women at large through literature, whilst discussing and sharing my own ideas. All of this studying was particularly encouraging and enlightening and set me on a path of exploration, which has continued until this day.

Now I can honestly say I have a passion for language, whether written or spoken and my relationship with the written or spoken word has taken me on a particularly fascinating journey. My work has extended me in ways that have been pleasantly surprising, travelling as far as the US and the Caribbean to promote/research intercultural dialogue, thereby sharing and developing creative ideas within a wider perspective.

I enjoy writing and editing and I write everyday, whether an article a blog or poetry. I love the elements of poetic rhythms; the voice, expression of feeling, use of imagination, thinking in images, dreaming and associating – all these aspects of creating my work have inspired me. I also love to read – my favourite author is Toni Morrison – my favourites from her collection are *Beloved* and *A Mercy*.

The personal essay genre is more than 400 years old and is one of my favourite ways to express honesty, the past, expansions of the self, and much more. It should certainly be celebrated, because it is one of the most approachable and diverting types of literature we possess. It possesses the freedom to move anywhere, in all directions. I have learned a lot from reading *The Art of the Personal Essay* by Phillip Lopate (recommended reading for personal essay enthusiasts).

* * *

Shangwe's website www.shangwe.com was created and launched in January 2005 with the main purpose of contributing to the development of new Black British literature by promoting writing by and for UK Black and Mixed-Race women. In this context, Shangwe aims to inform, inspire and empower these women writers, build their confidence and encourage their participation in the arts, and ensure that UK Black and Mixed-Race women's writing makes a historical literary contribution to Black British writing

In September 2008 and as part of Black History Month, I advertised for, collected and edited Black women's Africentric natural hair stories to post on a new blog. The aim was to provide an interactive dialogue of visual and written expressions to share our journeys to natural hair styles. What was profound for me was how much I enjoyed working with the mixed media of creative writing and photography, which has added a new dimension to my work.

A diverse range of hair stories and poems were received from ten contributors of African and African-Caribbean descent and these were published, one every three days, on blog www.hairjournal.blogspot.com, which was launched on 1st October 2008.

I discovered that black and mixed-race women had lots to say in their hair stories, which included, as was to be expected, the good, the bad and the ugly experiences they had encountered over the years, which had influenced them to finally aim for a more natural hair style.

In December 2008, I carried out an evaluation of the Hair Stories project and received positive feedback. For one contributor, writing her hair story was her first attempt at creative writing:

'This was my first creative piece and it was an extremely cathartic experience. I felt so at peace when I completed it. I wanted it to be poetic and yet provide a story about my life through the journey of my hair. This short piece prompted me to write a 4,000+ word short story using the themes from the short creative piece...' (Nehanda Buchanan, 22/12/08).

In particular, although many participants felt proud to see their written submissions published on-line, they thought the next stage would be to see their work in a printed format, i.e. a collection.

In May 2009, I returned to the project and decided to add the theme of skin so as to widen the project's scope for a potential anthology. The hair and skin themes are important to me for a number of reasons. For example, society, particularly the beauty and fashion industries still maintain a closed shop when it comes to the selection and promotion of models. In women's magazines, on catwalks, even shop dummies, dark skin is rarely seen. In this context, light skin and straight hair affirm superior human status.

* * *

The purpose of this collection is to offer the creative expressions of 48 Black and Mixed-Race women writers whose voices are among those defining this new era of contemporary Black British literature. The creative energies within this book offer a greater understanding and insight into creative writing by black and mixed-race women. In the pages that follow, you will read personal essays and poems that explore the issues, interests, cultural and historical influences that have shaped our times and our imaginations. The writers offer empowering, encouraging and creative ways of understanding and relating to the themes of hair and skin. The voices collected here range from teenage to mature, rural and urban, all contributing to this collection's diverse creativity.

My target was 40 writers, which I exceeded, and that is why I was pleased to include six writers based outside the UK – three from the US, one from Canada, one from Berlin and one from Botswana. I can thank my website for enabling this international opportunity to materialise.

Putting this book together has been an artistic experience merged with the business of publishing. Independently publishing this collection through Shangwe – separate from the mainstream – has been a great experience. I am not competing with publishers who mostly want to put books on shelves and see them fly off. I am promoting something new and rare.

One of the things that struck me as I was going through the process of putting this collection together is how wonderfully the selections work as a whole. It is evident that these writers have a common thread that extends beyond their fellowship as wordsmiths.

In my first Shangwe anthology *Brown Eyes*, I wrote 'my ambition is to produce another two titles, subject to funding...!' Well I'm pleased that I have achieved my ambition – however, it could never have happened without a host of talented writers, some previously unheard, some previously published, who share their individual voices and perspectives.

Fundamental to any collection is the contributors' participation and on this I am clear –a community of Shangwe writers has emerged - many have performed their contributions to my previous two anthologies at the Shangwe Poetry Events held between 2006 and 2008 at the Poetry Café, Covent Garden, London - thereby promoting Black and Mixed-Race women's writing adding a new dimension to UK Black literature.

Nicole Moore

HAIR POWER – SKIN REVOLUTION

HAIR STORIES

GROWING ROOTS

Patsy Antoine

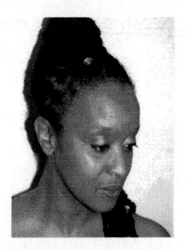

I hated my roots. I'm ashamed to admit it, but I did. Hated the kinky life they had of their own; the thick 'unmanageable' new growth; the bushy clumps that contrasted so dramatically with its straighter ends. You see straight was in. Nappy heads were out. So I'd willingly grown into despising my kink and convinced myself I was acceptable only if I mirrored the 'dream' – billboard images that left no room for tightly wound curls or afro textures.

I was already some way along my journey to the 'straight side'. But maintaining it wasn't easy. The hot comb had singed my ears. The relaxers burnt my scalp. But it was a small price to pay when my hair, pressed or chemically straightened, fell in thick waves around my face. When it settled around my shoulders and moved fluidly like long grass in the wind.

But then came the steam treatments, and six-weekly visits to stamp out those 'unsavoury' roots. "Don't tong too regularly", "Avoid too much heat". But with a thick and luscious head of straight hair I was invincible. What could a little heat do? So, I tonged and blow dried, pressed and hot combed. Avoid heat? Fat chance. It was too much to ask of anyone, much less me whose tomboy tendencies could barely manage the extra care needed to maintain my 'do'.

Inevitably, it wasn't long before those gloriously straight tresses became wispy and weak, before the dream became a nightmare and my visits to the hairdresser became few and far between. So, I cut my hair short. Boy short. Cut out the relaxers, the leisure curl perm. Suddenly, roots that were unmanageable and unsightly became healthy and shiny.

Suddenly, I realised that my hair looked unhealthy, not because of my roots, but because of its chemically weakened ends. I was a 'natural' and as my hair grew back I embraced my 'fro, two-strand twists, single plaits and cane rows. For the first time in my adult life, I enjoyed my hair. No, I lie. I loved my hair.

I didn't realise it at the time, but I was already contemplating locks. It starts so deep within, you're unaware it's there. It simmers gently on a low heat; splattering you with blobs of comprehension until eventually it bubbles to the surface and overtakes you. I started mine with a head full of china bumps. Leaving the salon that day I have never felt so powerful.

Nine years on I understand that my hair is so much more than decorative; it is the very thing that connects me to who I am. By embracing my roots I grow another set of roots into my history, my culture. I now realise that my hair carries the energy of my ancestors, it curls with life and vibrancy and its kink reflects the spring in my contented step.

HEAR MY LIFETIME HAIR JOURNEY

Nehanda Buchanan

I was born with a head free of chemicals, combs and conditioners; my hair naturally curled into a beautiful black shiny covering. It soon became pomades, hot combs warmed by the paraffin heater to remove all trace of its naturalness. My mother wanted a style that would curb an unruly mess. I would endure the burnt ears to have a creation that I could comb and flick through, much like my blond and brunette peers, fear of rain and water entering my recreational swim ruining its slick condition.

Then like the sunrise, the seventies arrived and a woman across the Atlantic revolutionised mine and so many sisters' crown and glory to create another story. We walked with pride as our hot combs were binned and replaced with combs of red green and black plastic and metal teeth, wooden crafted creations' artistry that remained a lasting legacy of freedom and liberation. My awakening journey truly began. *Thank you Angela.*

Bonding with my sister sibling, a natural born stylist, beautiful adornments of rows of plaits, sometimes braided or lengthened with extensions of synthetic that looked like my own and lasting for months, would be removed as it started to take a journey of its own.

I loved the attention received of gasping admiration for these unique and expressive twists. Travelling to Africa's continent in Senegal, the plaits were developed further into the crème de la crème of my hair expression; microscopic detail with shells, beads and coins to add the final touch – truly an African queen connected to a family left unintentionally hundreds of years ago. Welcome home child.

My daughters arriving showed me some new and original styles of their own.

The scissors intercepted throughout this journey at significant times. Sitting in a barber's chair I would receive from my opposite gender a quizzical and discomforting stare; what was my sister doing in here?

My shaven head the final result would then be coloured in coppers and reds and the comb replaced with a soft brush – complete ease and ready to please. Hairdressers completely redundant with me, why no perm, no tongs, no weave No, No, No........

Here we are now, my hair locked in a style deemed wayward, condemned, scorned and even criminalised in an island that waves its flag of Yellow, Green and Black. Oh their wearer's received such hatred and flack.

These beautiful knots completely freed me of combs and are replaced with fingers that manoeuvre every single strand within a god blessed locktitians hand. My shaved coloured head of five years ago now sits on my shoulder, carrying with it my stories of life changes, none more significant than the loss of the man, my father that assisted in my creation but also the glory of seeing my eldest and only son's graduation.

My adornment now covers the aids that assist my diminished hearing; vanity. Practicality or pride, my hair and its life journey continues with ultimate love and growth within and outside.

THE EVOLUTION OF MY HAIR

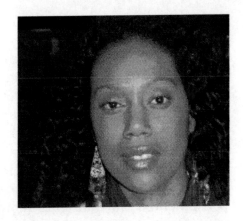

Monique Campbell

From plaits to cane rows to braids to hair-relaxers and then on to weaves – the journey of my hair seems never ending. Back in the day, prior to teeny-bop-hood, during the latter years of primary school when innocence still reigned upon me, having my hair divided in two to four sections used to be the 'lick'...well so my mother thought. I had long tresses of thick stranded semi-kinky hair that was marble-black and could locs with ease, which my mother found hard to manage. These two and four-sectioned partings of my hair where the tresses hung limp in my mother's hands and then transfixed into two or four plaits, were the repercussions of lacking time. And so I continued my primary school years with an inclination to learn how to groom my hair.

Teeny-bop-hood was infested with cravings for change: experimentation took centre-stage. I cane-rowed my hair backwards, frontwards, zigzags incorporated shapes that seemed for paper alone. I braided my hair thin, fat, with synthetic extensions, human extensions, no extensions. I cried experimentation, enjoyed the attention so much so that I dyed half my hair! The colour of the sun as it set upon the hilltop in *Sunset Beach*, still possessing my inherited frizz that *Dax* often shocked into waves.

My hair, I thought, was *the* coolest. Even when weave interfered with my natural long mane, luring me in with the prospect of wispy feathery European hair that moved airily in the wind and brushed across one's face, I thought I looked *the* coolest. I was edgy, had those funky cuts set on trend just like those commercial magazines displayed, except most of them did not reflect me. My decision to relax my hair was because I wanted to adopt this look permanently. Have my hair blowing in the wind as it did with the weave, but permanently.

With adulthood came again a time for change. I started to establish my identity, accept the things that made me, me. There were various contributing factors that drove me to my decision for this new type of change. One being that my hair was damaged and had lost its good quality and volume, the other being acceptance; the ability to accept the order and aesthetics of life, no matter which hand got dealt: dark-skin, light-skin, long-hair, short-hair, broad-nose, thin-nose, straight-hair or afro-hair. Ageing is unstoppable as are the seasons that follow one another, unfaltering in their existence.

I currently stand at a cross-road between principles and the dictatorship of time. At the age of 26 with seven willing years of strenuous management and gregarious results of natural hair under my belt, I am contemplating texturising. Not because I want to aspire to look like someone else or I'm unable to accept the natural conditions of my hair, but because I'm unable to provide my hair with the time it needs.

No longer do I have those spare 4-6 hours to wash, condition and twist my hair every two-weeks so that it looks presentable. My hair comes down to the centre of my back, can easily make three sets of heads and has curls that locs with ease. So my question is this: do I pander to my principles of acceptance? Or do I bow down to the dictatorship of time and put a solution in my hair that will merely loosen the curls and make it easier to manage whilst keeping the natural look (as put by my hairdresser *From the Roots*)?

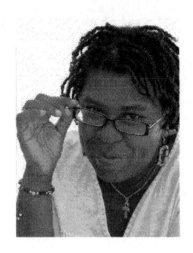

LIFETIME OF HAIR

Christine Collymore

Part One

As a child, my hair was mine but not under my control. I have pictures of me with an inch of afro, then hair straight with big ribbons. As long as I can remember, my hair has always been short, thick, and kinky. 'The hair hard'; 'Why you don't have pretty hair'; 'Oh gosh, you break another comb', were phrases that were trotted out every now and then. There were no positive comments, considering it was supposed to be my crowning glory. So I always saw my hair as a problem, something that had to be 'managed'. And managed it was, by the use of the hot comb. Then my hair became longer, less coarse and easy to put into a ponytail. I could have hairstyles like my school friends...

Part Two

...Now I have control of my hair and mind. And, yes, I went through the journey of continuing to 'manage' my hair with the use of chemicals, relaxers and curly perms. At the time, it didn't matter about the damage I was doing to my scalp; after all, 'no beauty without pain'. The phrases of 'nappy hair', 'It is a pity that you don't have good hair', still haunt and anger me.

I have learnt that I can undo the socialisation, which has affected my attitude and thoughts about my natural hair. I have experimented with twists, cornrows and my favourite, my afro. It is **my** crowning glory and I feel that I no longer have to look European to be proud of myself. In fact, I feel like a beautiful black woman of African and Caribbean descent living in England. What I love about my hair is the ability to be creative and be individual. What is it about the desire to touch an afro, got one message for you, look but don't touch?

I would consider locs, but I think that will be a story for part three.

MY JOURNEY....TO ME

Anduosjahla James-Wheatle

Reflection

It's a Sunday morning and my mother is greasing and combing my hair, one plait at the front, and two bunches at the back. Any distasteful noises which I made were met with extra tugging on the hair or a chop on my greased head with the comb!!! There was no scope to make demands on how I wanted my hair to be styled, it was washed, greased and styled to my mother's specification.

My father was a Rastafarian, and I know that he had explored the idea of me also growing locks, however he came up against some resistance from my mother. Given that I was an unconventional teenager who questioned 'why', albeit in a polite and respectful way, I developed a strong sense of affinity with feminism. I expressed a desire to grow locks; however my mother's response remained identical and consistent, with the response my father had received several years before. **The seed is planted...**

Experimentation

As I progressed through the experimental processes during my teenage years, I felt a great sense of relief when I finally obtained my mother's permission, to relax my hair. I thought this would be easier to maintain, grow longer, flow freely and be socially acceptable, which was a classic expectation at that age. To some extent it was easier to maintain, but the need for length and flow in a vertical direction were realistically unobtainable.

The experiment began: the gels and relaxers were utilised, as well as many different colours, high top weaves and extensions; no distance was too far for me to travel, in order for me obtain 'my' look. This was all about me receiving acknowledgement, but always with the recognition that I was unique and different to everybody else, so my hair style had to be a direct reflection of me. I became bored, I knew the chemicals were no good for my hair, nevertheless I persevered. I longed to grow locks, and constantly expressed my need to make that decision, parallel to a sense of anxiety and sense of acceptance. **Distinction...or was it?**

Spiritual direction

I stood in the mirror one day in September 2008, at approximately 1am in the morning and chopped.... and chopped, the relaxed, tired and processed hair. There I was looking back at me, a face I hadn't seen for over 15 years, it was the natural me, natural beauty.

It was time, I had received a wink from God, and He was guiding me through this next phase. Nothing happens by coincidence, and it was far bigger than a 'style' or 'look'. All the concerns and worries which I had were insignificant; this was the 'I' which was waiting to emerge. Now I have locks, my hair is the shortest it has ever been and I feel liberated, beautiful and have a sense of freedom. I've started my journey... **Patience**

NB 'Dread'- Fear, Terror, Horror: I do not have dreadlocks, I have 'locks' as I do not identify my locks with the description given above, neither are they intended to give that impression to others.

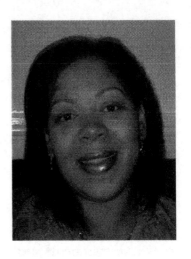

NATURALLY RELAXED!

Colette Machado

The transition from having relaxed hair to going natural was interestingly made in a very natural way (excuse the pun). For almost 15 years I relaxed my hair on average about twice a year to get that dead straight, silky look, which of course I was not born with. Yes, after years of enduring those burning sensations at each relaxing session, it is hard to believe that the decision to go natural was so easy. Gosh, wouldn't it be great if making decisions generally was as easy as this?

OK, let me confess. If I am to be honest I did not really make a decision to go natural, the decision was made for me, knowing that it was the right thing to do. Also, there was no plan to go natural or stay natural, again this too happened naturally and without even thinking "should I", "shouldn't I", etc.

So, why and when did I decide to go au naturel? It was January 2005; the start of a New Year and half-way into the month when I found out that I was pregnant. Totally overjoyed, I wanted to do everything right; find out as much information as I could about pregnancy, the development of the baby, etc. My maternal instincts were kicking in and I felt an overwhelming desire to protect my unborn child.

Soon after, I remember thinking to myself hmmm, is relaxing my hair actually safe for the baby? After all, I am putting chemicals into my hair...so could they pass through to the baby I wondered? Some people may call me neurotic for thinking this, and why did I not think the same way about deodorants that I sprayed on my body passing through to the baby too but the strong smell of the relaxer and the ingredients in it is enough to tell you why!

Research told me that no evidence to date proved that the chemicals in relaxers were harmful to a growing baby in the womb but there was also no evidence that proved that it wasn't! The general printed advice (across several books/magazines) leaned towards the fact that when pregnant, women should refrain from putting chemicals in their hair to be on the safe side. I too decided to go down this road – and have gladly never looked back.

I did not plan to stay natural. When my hair was next due for relaxing after giving birth to my son, as a busy mum, the trip to the hairdressers kept being put off and off, and it continued like this until I questioned whether in fact my hair really needed relaxing after all. The clear answer to this was 'no'.

The great thing is that after having natural hair for almost four years I do not regret the decision to go or stay natural one bit. My hair is still easy to manage, style, look after, etc, and in its natural state is in fact much healthier, since I've stopped relaxing it, stronger and the length it was before I relaxed it.

In fact I have never looked back, and I truly hope I never will. Why would I want to tamper with my natural hair state....when there is not a thing wrong with it? As the saying goes, if it ain't broke, don't fix it!

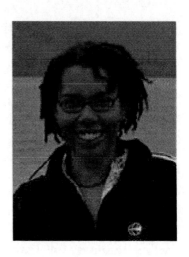

I'VE GOT 'GOOD' HAIR

Sheree Mack

"You've got good hair!" A constant chorus fed to me by my family as I was growing up. With this exclamation the customary feel of my hair would follow, just to make sure. My hair was 'good' because it was thick but also straight and not so 'kinky'. I was told I had the best hair in the family and should feel lucky. I really didn't feel lucky. I always had to wear my hair in plaits or bunches, with ribbons and bobbles. I could never wear my hair out and down. Why? Because, it could never withstand the elements. Rain or wind, my hair would become a tangled knotty shrunk mess.

I thought I could change this with a perm. My mum let me. I went to the local hairdressers in Newcastle, meaning I was the first black head they got their hands on. The hairdresser said she'd have to straighten my hair first and then perm it, because it was so strong. This was my first time in a real hairdressers and I think the experience went to my head literally, because when she asked me if I wanted it cut, I just said, 'Yes, go for it.' I wanted the glamour – I wanted long straight hair that I could only achieve when I had a large towel on my head with the folds cascading down my back.

The hairdresser straightened, permed and layered my hair. That was over 20 years ago and my hair hasn't been the same since. Something must have gone wrong in the process because it looked 'good' when it was wet. This was my 'wet look' phase. My hair was constantly wet; dripping wet, and gelled up to the nines. I got a fringe from that trip to the hairdressers, a fringe I treated like gold dust. I pulled and curled it with curling tongs. I had to be more careful though, after I burnt my forehead. My god that hurt! I've still got the scar.

I hated washing my hair, as afterwards I'd spend the whole week pulling and brushing my hair until it came out, stretched out of its tight curls into loose curls. By the time it was back to a decent length it would be time to wash it again. There's something wrong when you feel that your hair is 'good' when it's dirty.

Then when I became a mother, entering a new phase in my life, I had all my 'good' hair chopped off. I became peanut head, as my husband named me. It was basically a skin-head look with my fringe still, which revealed to me that I had a small head and a beautiful profile. I enjoyed this phase of my life as I could just wash and go. I enjoyed the freedom, even though while teaching, I got called 'Sonique' by the school kids.

Then there was the time that I got locked extensions put in, but that's a whole other story. Now, my hair is locked naturally. I didn't go the hairdressers – not after my earlier experiences. Most days I wear my hair out and down, and it's glorious because it stays put against the rain and the wind. I run my fingers through it and it feels good. That's 'good' hair.

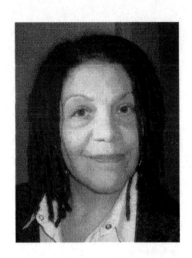

A JOURNEY TO NATURAL HAIR

Nicole Moore

When I reflect back to the time when I felt the most natural and free-spirited it was the seventies and eighties when I wore an afro hairstyle. There was no need to spend endless hours at a hairdressers – the thought never entered my head. With the minimum of fuss, my natural hair grew free and all I used in between weekly washes was an Afro comb, *Vaseline* hair lotion and oil sheen on my tresses. I kept my hair in this natural style for many years.

Fast forward to the twenty-first century and like most women, I have been influenced by fashion trends from the likes of Jjeri curl, which meant my hair grew lengthways and soon reached my shoulders, braid extensions which kept the long hair look that I liked but didn't last for longer than a couple of months, and relaxing, which I now realise was the most unnecessary, hazardous and risky route my hair embarked upon. A breakthrough came when I discovered that instead of such a harsh way to straighten my hair, I could blow dry my hair instead of resorting to using chemicals.

I think experimenting with different styles in the pursuit of fashion can be creative as you explore different looks. However, hair and identity are intrinsically linked – whether you think you are just wearing a hair style – your hair style does say something about you.

It has been over three years since I last combed my hair. In September 2006, after a lot of thought and consideration, I decided to embark upon locsing my hair. I remember my first visit to the locs hairdressers was much more than an appointment. As I sat discussing this next stage of my return to natural hair with my loctitian, the scenario around me of women and men who were getting their beautiful locs re-twisted and styled was enough to inspire and reinforce my decision to locs my hair. There is no doubt about it, many black and mixed-race women are embracing their natural hair with pride, and challenging those Eurocentric fashion trends that seek to influence their lives. They are discovering that black hair is beautiful left to its own devices.

I never intended my locs to be a fashion statement. I was returning full circle to an authentic and liberating hair style. It was a commitment – a natural and cultural expression of pride in my ethnicity first and foremost.

Author, Alice Walker, who has worn her hair in locs since the eighties, once wrote, 'Bob Marley is the person who taught me to trust the universe enough to respect my hair; as he shook his lion's mane, the confidence, the love, and the sheer commitment to Blackness and to Jah was in his every moment.'

Three years on and I still love my locs and it is difficult to imagine myself without them. They are here to stay as they are connected not only to my head but also to my African-Caribbean cultural heritage and history. However, having said that, they mean less to me in terms of Rastafarianism – although I respect Rastafarian beliefs – and more in terms of spiritual and personal freedom. Wearing locs is a way of freeing me both figuratively and literally from the dictates of western European fashion.

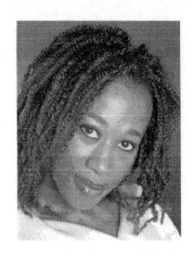

HAIR TO STAY

Brenda White

I could think of so many hair stories. It's been really hard choosing which story to share. I could tell you about the stories of having my hair washed as a child, and how much I hated it, or even the dreaded anticipation I had when my mum would practically rake the comb through my hair that was left uncombed for days.

Yes... I have had my ups and downs with my hair just like everyone else. I have tried various styles and textures over the years from cornrows and braiding to relaxing.

Relaxing required regular maintenance, and is not surprising when you think of the chemical contents. At least once a month I would go to the hairdressers for a steam and maybe have the ends clipped to stop split ends. This would set me back at least fifty pounds.

I would spend a fortune to look beautiful and groomed, especially when it came to my hair. My hair did look good, but there was no way I could keep this up forever. I wondered what my hair would look like if I stopped relaxing it. 'You will have to cut it out gradually or it will break', my hairdresser advised me.

Eleven years ago while pregnant, I made the decision that I wanted my hair natural, maybe even locks. My influence had come from an understanding of myself and my culture. This included music influences, for example, Bob Marley, Burning Spear, and my visits to the Caribbean.

I was now 35 and I wanted a new look. Then it dawned on me that my hair was part of my uniqueness. My new look would now represent me and my heritage. I concluded that my hair was my connection to my people. Anywhere in the world I saw people with hair like mine, I knew that they were connected to me and the African Diaspora.

Africans are the only race with tightly curled hair. I read that it is like this to keep us cool in the hot sun of the African continent. To me, it helps us to stand out as a nation. We may be some of the most deprived people in the world, but our presence can never be denied.

It took me years to come to my decision and I am glad that I did. I am proud of my blackness and I wear my hair in many beautiful natural styles, mainly afro; a style that stood for liberation for black people back in the seventies. I wear my hair with pride and as a continuation of one of the physical traits of my people.

PERSONAL ESSAYS: HAIR

"Black women straighten their hair because we are told, probably by someone who is not Black, that our hair should be straight. Although this defies everything we are or hope to be, we do it to the tune of six billion dollars every year."

'The Value in the Valley', Iyanla Vanzant (1995)

AFRO CHIC

Louisa Adjoa-Parker

When I was little, I was a bit puzzled about the springy substance that grew upwards from my head, instead of downwards like it did with my friends. All of my life I've lived in mainly white areas and my relationship with my hair has been affected by this. I'd have given anything to have long, blonde, straight hair that swung like a silky curtain when I moved my head, hair that I could flick back flirtatiously. Instead, I had a ball of frizz sitting on top of my head, much like, as I was constantly told, a brillo pad.

When my Ghanaian father still lived with us, he did my hair. I remember the smell of the hair dressing he used, in a little red tin, and having my hair regularly trimmed into a short, neat afro – not one of the funky seventies' afros that people on TV wore. Occasionally, my white English mum would put my hair into braids, like fat snakes, with beads on the ends. I hated this – it was too 'African' and I was busy trying to blend chameleon-style into my white environment, which was no easy task.

Other children would ask to touch my hair, and then comment freely on what they thought it felt or looked like. This ranged from sheep's wool and cotton wool, through to 'Looking as though I'd had an electric shock'. And how can

I forget the 'Ooh, it's like pubes' wisecracks? I'd shrug all of this off; after all, I had heard it hundreds of times during my childhood. But of course it hurt, and my relationship with my hair and identity as a mixed heritage child was damaged.

My dad left when I was 13, and we moved to Devon from East Anglia. As a teenager, hair is a huge part of your identity, and I found this stage of my life especially hard. My mum did not know what to do with it, so tried to keep up the family tradition of short afros. But I was turning into a young woman and hated having short hair – it was too masculine. I got my ears pierced and wore dangly earrings, so at least they would flap about prettily in the breeze, even if my hair didn't.

We had no hair products, and even if we'd known of their existence, wouldn't have been able to buy them in Devon, where there were no other black people to be seen. I had grown up with simply no knowledge of African-Caribbean hair styling. Apart from my emotionally absent father in the early years of my life, I grew up around white people, who didn't teach me how to do my hair; their only contribution hair-wise was to teach me how to hate it.

One distressing memory sticks in my mind. When I was 14, my afro was rebelling against my parent's version of a basin hair-cut and doing its best to grow. One day my mum got angry after I'd gone AWOL for a few hours. She threw me into a chair, shouting that I looked like a tramp, and cut most of my hair off. I felt so ugly and masculine, but still had to go to school the following Monday with a shorn head. I was trying to be feminine and attractive, and here I was with stubby, frizzy hair framing what I thought was an ugly, round face.

In the late eighties, big hair was in fashion, so I managed to dodge the afro-shearing sessions and grow my hair as much as it could grow. I tried to create a 'fringe' by constantly pulling my hair down in front of my eyes. I wanted to be able to peer out behind a curtain of hair that grew into my kohl-lined eyes. I didn't quite achieve the look I was going for – it was more afro-quiff than New Romantic fringe. Later I got a hot brush, the eighties equivalent of GHDs, and used this to straighten my hair. I refused to go anywhere without it. My white friends found this hilarious, but I just wanted to be like the people around me. I lived in constant fear of rain, as my hair mysteriously shrunk when it came into contact with water, even when I had not straightened it. After this I went through a 'hippy' phase, and braided my hair, then let it turn into dreads. I'd experiment by bleaching and dying my hair bright colours. The result was an orangey mass of matted hair. Still, it was (minimally) better than a boyish afro.

When I had my first child, I decided I should look more respectable so I cut most of my dreads off, although I couldn't let go of a few at the front of my head, thus creating a 'dreaded' fringe. I eventually pulled these out, grew my hair and began to wear it in a bun, like a rabbit's tail on the top of my head. I first discovered hair relaxer when I went to Switzerland to visit my sister. She booked a hair appointment with a stressed-out woman at the end of her working day, who not only didn't protect my hair but also didn't tell me how to look after it. I loved the look of my newly-softened curls when wet, and washed my hair every day that hot summer. With no products to condition it, inevitably it broke and I had to use hair grips to clip up the stumpy strands.

I began to learn about black hair products, but still didn't know where to get them, apart from Switzerland. Later, I had an Ethiopian friend who could occasionally be persuaded to braid my hair when I went to visit her in London. We'd sit in her living room, talking and smoking cigarettes into the early hours to get it done. It was not until I was in my thirties that I found a hairdresser locally (thirty miles away) that could cater for my hair. I was so happy, and had my first ever haircut by a hairdresser, and tried weaves and braids. I was really upset when she, rather selfishly I thought, decided to have a baby and stop hairdressing!

Last year I had a weave-on-from-hell disaster when I went to a woman in Exeter. The weave was put in so tightly it pulled some of my hair out, and even more came out when she yanked the weave out and then proceeded to burn my hair with the hottest, most smoke-inducing hairdryer I've ever seen. I bought a European wig, which set me back £150. I felt so fake, sticking it on my head every morning and was terrified it would blow off in a strong wind. I found a less hair-yanking hairdresser in Southampton and had another weave. After this my hair grew back and I was relieved to no longer see patches of skin where my hair had once been.

My hair has been a massive problem: how society and I see it, and what to do with it. Now I'm growing it out after having it texturised and it breaking, yet again. My fiancé loves my natural hair, and this helps me to accept it more. Some of my friends tell me they have always preferred my natural hair, but I just was not listening to them at the time, so caught up was I in the idea that it was 'wrong'. I have always seen my hair through European eyes, and I want to change that. I was not born with straight hair so why should I sew other people's hair onto my head? Why should I put toxic chemicals on my scalp to destroy the natural texture of my hair? The view that straight hair is beautiful is not the only view – there is more than one type of beauty.

It's interesting that I feel differently about my hair in different places. In rural Dorset where I live now, my hair is so different to European hair and stands out like a beacon. Yet when I go to London or other urban areas I feel self-conscious for a different reason – I feel I look poor and uncared for with my natural, chemically damaged hair. I feel like a country bumpkin who has just got off the train with a piece of grass hanging out of my mouth. So, nowhere do I feel I really fit in. This is something I'm having to learn in my late thirties – to feel that I fit in with others as well as feeling at home in my own skin (or hair).

I'm still wearing hair-pieces and straightening my hair, while it's growing out. And then I want to learn how to style my natural hair in a way that won't damage it. I'm learning to like this kinky, frizzy mop, and hope this is the beginning of a beautiful friendship.

TAMING THOSE TRESSES

Natalie Ambersley

Growing up I dreamed of having long, poker straight hair that laid flat and never moved even in the strongest of winds! Being born of mixed race heritage I was born with the complete opposite: big, thick flyaway hair that curled at every opportunity, regardless of whether I straightened with hot irons or slept in one of those unattractive hair nets! I will always remember as a little girl, when my mum would sit me down in between her legs every morning before school, battling with my hair, combing it, greasing it and making sure it was tightly pulled into a secure bun without a single strand out of place. Endless tears were shed as she tried to comb out all the knots from the day before, which was made increasingly worse after a night tossing and turning in my sleep.

When I came of age and was old enough to take on the responsibility of taming my own tresses, my mum was more than happy to place the afro comb securely into the hands of its new owner: Me. The result of this natural transition was that I was now spending numerous mornings crying into the mirror because my hair was big, curly and never styled the way I wanted it to. Growing up in a predominantly white area, all my friends had straight, free flowing blond hair and that's what I wanted, not a huge pile of frizzy curls that resembled the likes of Diana Ross during her Supreme days. Every morning, I would pile on *Soft 'n' Free, Dark and Lovely,* or anything I could find that promoted "controlling your curls". And it didn't matter how much I piled it on, nothing seemed to work on my stubborn mane! All I wanted was flat, lifeless hair like my white friends (sorry girls!), and trying to obtain that look was impossible.

Then one day I discovered the relaxer kit, which to me sounded like a miracle invention. 'Great' I thought as I made my way down East Ham High street in search of a relaxer kit, which I thought would be the answer to all my hair troubles. Finally, a product that would give me straight hair like I had dreamed of, accept it wasn't to be. As I massaged the solution into my scalp, the strong peroxide smell wafting up my nostril along with the burning sensation that instantly kicked in, I questioned how damaging this was to my hair. Nevertheless, that didn't stop me buying one relaxer kit after the other.

By the time the process was complete all my curls had disappeared and there I was with lovely straight hair that I could flick from one side to the other like the girls out of *Baywatch*! However, because luck wasn't on my side, the next morning there would be a sudden heavy downpour of rain, and with an umbrella unable to save me, my hair would be back to its normal curly self. Moisture in the air, humidity or a tiny speckle of rain would send my hair into an uncontrollable frenzy.

I've gone from relaxers, curly perms, plaits to weaves, all in a desperate bid to make me feel happy and confident with my hair. So my next drastic move after the relaxer was simple. I went for the chop. By cutting my hair shorter, I thought I would be cutting away the curls for good. However, going for the scissors made no difference, the dreaded curl was still there ingrained into my scalp, and I was still reduced to tears every time I looked in the mirror and wondered what I was going to do with it next?

Now a distant memory, I look back wondering why I made such a big fuss about having curly hair, as these days I love nothing more than having big, bouncy curls. I opt for a very natural look, which evolved after educating myself on how mixed race hair is supposed to be. Celebrities such as Angela Griffin, Melanie Brown, and Leona Lewis all opt for the natural look and in effect have helped me to love my hair.

My style is simple yet effective. Brown curls with light blonde and golden brown highlights and I love it! Like most women, I still have bad hair days when I look in the mirror and think *you are a mess*, but to be honest those days of hating my hair are well and truly behind me. I spend most mornings trying to make my hair look bigger, rather than trying to make it look as flat as cardboard! For me, it's a case of the bigger it is, the more confident I feel. The general assumption with such a style is that I must be bold and confident if I can wear my hair so dramatically, none of which is true. I just like to be a bit different and not succumb to the norm. So it's no more relaxers or hair dryers for me, just a natural bounce that I wouldn't swap for anything. People often say, "You always want what you can't have" but when it comes to my hair I couldn't be happier!

MY BAD HAIR LIFE

Catherine Anthony Boldeau

In its natural state, I have the kind of 'Negro' hair that only true 'niggers' possess. If my ancestors mated with Orientals, Asians or European's there's little evidence of this in my appearance. I'm just black! My skin is chocolate brown, velvety smooth and translucent. My hair is coarse, tight and curly. It is reminiscent of a steel brillo pad, only prettier. My coal curls endemic of my African heritage. Only most Africans I know have softer, more manageable locks.

I've often wondered where my ancestors came from, but as I haven't taken the trouble to seriously trace my genealogy, except back two generations, there is little to go on. Apparently, my maternal great-grandfather was white and my paternal grandmother had long Asian hair. But these discoveries make me none the wiser about why my hair has such an outstanding criminal record.

Throughout my life my hair has been so out of control that it has received several anti-social behaviour orders. It assaults comb after comb. Several macho rakes suffer grievous bodily harm and are reduced to the plastic recycle bin, after spending only a few moments in my "coco rolls", the affectionate name given to my hair by my Asian

Caribbean husband, who prides himself that his straight hair is somehow superior to mine.

My hair has been incarcerated on numerous occasions for being 'drunk and disorderly' after guzzling tub after tub of afro hair conditioning sheen, more commonly known as "grease"; graduating from the "lite" conditioning moisturising cream to the "strong stuff" for dry, dull and lifeless hair. It's taken me years to dry out. And, believe me, even today at the age of 40, after nearly two decades of rehab, I am only one step away from my next crisis.

My bad hair life started in January 1972 at the age of five, just around the time I started school and Grandma died. Like mother, I thought granny would live forever. Grandma was a small, yet strong ebony lady with a sweet broad smile that matched the warmth of her huge heart. She was always nicely dressed, even at home and she took great care of all her hairpieces and wigs, so that she looked immaculate.

Apparently, when I was two, she saved my poor little arse from a beating by my father. My mother tells me that I was an adventurous toddler who had ideas that were far above my height and station. Not satisfied to stay on the ground, I used the available chairs and our rickety old dining table as my Mount Everest.

My father, terrified that I might not soar to the heights that I wished to attain tried to smack me for my childish attempts at mountaineering. He saw my infantile scheme to reach the summit as an act of defiance. So, when he entered the dining room with that deep large scowl on his face, his large hands poised to connect with my behind, I knew I was in a for a good hiding. My Bible-believing grandmother instantly became my saviour as she placed herself between Eustace Nathaniel Anthony and me and prevented him from committing a certain act of violence.

"Stacey, in your wrath, remember mercy," she said.

Her knowledge of scripture had the desired effective.

My guilt-ridden father lowered his hand and slunk away with his head down. I repeated grandma's words to daddy the next day, when once again, I tried to scale the heights of our cluttered dining room. It worked. My grandmother's lesson was learnt early – the word of the Lord could certainly change things – well, my father at least.

Grandma was truly a saint. Her generosity knew no bounds. You only had to turn up on her doorstep and you would be fed and watered. And no one ever left granny's house without at least a bag of groceries.

"Take a little something, just in case you can't go shopping", she would say in her mellow Trinidadian brogue. I believe that the only reason that the good Lord took her when He did was that she needed some much-deserved rest.

The death of my grandmother deeply affected my mother's life. She had put adulthood on hold while her mother was alive and now she needed a dummy to practise on. So I became her black *Barbie* doll.

Each Sunday afternoon, my mother would shampoo my hair without any conditioner. At the end of each washing session, the torture phase began; the pulling and tugging reminiscent of a prolonged lynching, only worse. My mother's hands ripped through my tender scalp sending layer on layer of pain ice-skating through my cerebrum, actuating somersaults over my neck and performing the foxtrot with sensuous abandon up and down the length of my spine.

"Keep still", she bellowed, "I'm not hurting you".

Like hell, you weren't! "Soon I will be done a wid the trouble of de worl". This Mahalia Jackson spiritual spoke volumes to me. Throughout my ordeal, dripping towels, irritating combs, a throbbing head and an aching heart, I whimpered. Like a blind bloodhound, on the verge of entering doggy heaven with the prospect of frisky chattering poodles as your only champion for eternity.

I paid handsomely for my rebellion. Mother interpreted my wriggling as a gross act of disobedience.

"Disobedience was the first sin," she would scream.

"You know that the wages of sin is death."

I would have rather faced death for it was tug after tug of war. I always ended up the loser with a tear-streaked face and a world-weary soul after several hours of drying and plaiting.

When I was five, mother plaited my hair twice; first, in about 30 or so small knots before re-plaiting in two very tight cornrows. After years of trying to make cornrows, a full-head plait, I can't make my attempts look even slightly credible. My mother, however, has perfected this hairdressing technique and regularly chides me, "You still can't do hair".

My mother's cornrows lasted six days. On the seventh day, instead of resting, like the Good Book recommends, my hair was mercilessly tied in two pigtails that resembled horns. Each one emblazoned with matching ribbons of varying sizes, colours and textures – whatever matched my Sabbath best.

My mother has kept the washed out orange shoe box filled with the wilted ribbons, bands and cacophony of other old-fashioned hair accessories from a bygone age. She is proud of this heirloom and is determined to pass it to my dual heritage five year old.

"Why don't you put ribbons in Arianne's hair?"

She threw the words into conversation recently. Age has not lessened her insistence and she cut through me with those diamond sharp eyes that even the onset of cataracts can't diminish.

"I'll give you some."

She's persistent.

"Why am I the only person who makes Arianne's hair look nice?"

I dismiss her.

My mother's sense of self-righteous indignation is evident when I blatantly refuse the repulsive container and its appalling contents. Her anger was never so distinguished as when she would spy the "unribboned" heads of my friends in church whose "mothers simply can't be bothered to make their daughters look respectable in the House of God".

I, however, came to envy Kim, Donna, Janet, Stephanie, Denise, Delcina and Marina for their ribbon-free hairstyles. To mother, ribbons and hair bands symbolise femininity in a bygone colonist age, of blameless motherhood and moral Christian behaviour.

Because of my mother's constant nagging about my looks and the awful things I should put in my hair, I started to imagine I was a boy; a trouser-wearing *Tony* with short neat hair and commanding looks. As young as I was, there was something inside me that resisted her opaque female mind.

I was never going to be a black Scarlett O'Hara, decked out in lace and ribbons, fainting at the sight of the lack of respectability, fanning wildly, pretending to be the epitome of modesty and meekness, sitting in the "House of the Lord on the Lord's Day", all tightly corseted and stringed, "rejoicing in Jesus", with a fake smile to match my false spirituality. Nor was I going to pretend to be an Aunt Jemima, with the hand-me down identity, in those old black and white movies. I wanted someone to say to me, "You'll be a man, my son". But there was no Rudyard Kipling to encourage me. I was the product of my mother and grandmother. I was reluctantly feminine, with my "coal curls" and "ink imagination". I was Woman. I am Black Woman.

HAIR: A JOURNEY OF SELF DISCOVERY

Scherin Barlow Massay

My hair was first straightened on the eve of me travelling to England to join my parents. My grandmother woke me up early that morning and took me to the home of a neighbour who lived a few doors away. On the back porch, an array of buckets had been filled with water. Washing outside was not unusual, because in the hot climate of Guyana, it was normal for children to be bathed outside in the evenings instead of being showered indoors. But what was unusual was that it was day-time and someone, apart from a family member was doing the washing.

My hair was washed several times, conditioned with okra leaves, and dried. It was parted into sections, greased and straightened with a pair of pressing combs, as I sat on the porch, being cooled by the morning breeze. Afterwards, I remember looking into a mirror and admiring my new straight style. Although the process had been painful and I was still smarting from a burnt scalp, I felt proud at my initiation into the grown-up world of women. Most girls my age would have had to wait until their late teens before that "Rights of Passage" was bestowed upon them, usually in preparation for a first date or job interview. My hair was then put into rollers made from twisted newspaper, which was secured around each small parting and left to set until the next day. However, when I awoke the next morning, to my shame and everyone else's horror, my hair had reverted back to its natural state as though the last twenty-four hours had been completely obliterated!

In my teens, I didn't bother too much with my hair because socialising in the form of partying was not on my list of priorities. My laissez-faire attitude towards my hair meant that I kept it plaited. However, when I did go out, it was kept under a wrap. Head wrapping had become symbolic of a conscious recognition of an African identity amongst some African Caribbean young women. And it was also the continuation of the Caribbean tradition of wearing a head tie, albeit, in a different style. The head tie (traditionally worn by older women) was a square, folded into a triangle; whereas, the wrap was a long rectangular piece of cloth, custom made by the individual.

In my twenties, I started partying and soon realised that pressed hair and sweaty environments did not mix! After crawling out of a shebeen, in the early hours of the morning, the last thing I wanted was pressed hair that had shrivelled up and reverted back to its natural state, like Cinderella's carriage! Therefore, a chemical relaxer seemed like the perfect solution to the problem. For a few weeks after relaxing my hair, it looked lovely. It could be styled the way I wanted, with curls cascading from the top. However, I also suffered the indignities of hair that fell out, and on many occasions, I sported hair that could only be slicked back into a Bessie Smith type hair style because it was too short for anything else. But although my scalp received chemical burns and my hair was left damaged, I continued the practice of relaxing my hair for many years.

Today, my hair has been chemically-free for more than 15 years. One sunny day, I decided to pay homage to the naturalness of my hair; so with an afro, picked out to the fullest, I made my way to East London's Ridley Road Market to shop and gauge the reaction on people's faces. Many of the women (all wearing weaves), looked at me briefly, before turning away. I could see embarrassment etched on their faces. Had I exposed their secret? Or were they feeling sorry for me, believing that I had lost the plot?

In the market, a man came up to me and commented that he had seen me on the main road but he was in his car. 'My hair?' I asked. He replied, 'Yes! It looks lovely and you look so confident.' With a twinkle in my eye, I smiled at him and replied 'Freedom'. He nodded and I went away thinking that he was a man who had not lost his real sense of identity; one who was not fooled by what society dictates.

My emancipation did not come about from a Eurocentric perspective. Rather, I had to educate myself from an African viewpoint. This quest that first began in my teens, really found its groundings when I went to university. There, I was shocked and delighted to discover that a Caribbean Centre had recently been set up as one of the university's educational faculties. I quickly attached myself to the Centre; working for two terms as part of my coursework and voluntarily for the duration of my studies as part of my own programme for self development. The Centre began to open up a new world of knowledge for me. It had a library filled with books that I never knew existed. I read books on socio-linguistics from an African-Caribbean perspective. I read books on the customs of the Caribbean, tracing their roots back to Africa. I learnt the reasons behind the social and economic conditions that persist in Africa and the Caribbean. I read and researched anything that took my interest. The person appointed to develop the Caribbean Centre, quickly became my mentor and friend. Many of the courses she developed were taught by academics who like her, were from the African diaspora.

I attended lectures that left me on academic highs for days. And as my knowledge increased, I eagerly began to reconstruct a new identity, one that was firmly grounded in my roots as an African, born in the diaspora.

What did I mean when I made the comment about freedom? I meant that reconstructing an intact African identity had set me free from the pressures to conform to European stereotypes by my own people and those outside of my race. I meant that I was proud of my heritage and happy to embrace the real concept of beauty within my racial identity.

My preferred style is cornrows. I love that my hair can be made into such intricate styles that reflect and complement my ethnicity. I love to see the natural swirls and waves that come with naturally short textured hair.

But the main reason for me loving my hair natural is because I am happy living in the castle that is my skin and because I have an African-centric model of beauty that could never be erased from my mind.

UNWRITTEN RULES

Christine Collymore

It was a Sunday, my hair needed washing, so I decided not to undo the twists first. I gave my scalp a good massage with a well known shampoo and made sure that there was plenty of lather. When I had finished rinsing, my hair glistened, thankfully with the majority of twists still in place. All I had to do now was to towel dry, add some hair and scalp treatment and I was ready to go.

The rest of Sunday was filled with the delights of going out for a walk, visiting friends and family. Towards the end of the day, I started thinking about the rest of the working week and the meeting arranged on Monday. I went through the ritual of deciding what clothes I would be wearing, even managed to match shoes. All I had to do was sort out my hair. My hair looked like a mixed bag of sweets, there were some frizzy twists, some twisted to the end and others not. My hair did not look disgusting but the thought of going to the meeting like this did not sit well with me. I suppose the question is: why not?

I had choices. I could redo my hair, but that would take hours as the twists are portioned in small sections. Or I could wrap it; the problem was the weather for Monday forecasted a warm day, and having a black wrap covering my head would make me too hot. I could undo the hair and wear it in an afro, however, the issue now was I had just changed my hair from an afro style to twists. The main reason for the change was sustaining the level of maintenance required to keep my afro looking good. I was in no mood to go back to that in this hot weather and busy schedules. My final resort and option was to reach for the hair straightener. This would take about ten minutes and my hair would be sleek, shiny and no frizz.

On Monday morning I put on my earrings and lipstick, patted down my hair and I was ready to go. There was no thought about wanting long hair or wanting to look European. My hair was still natural, no chemicals, in the twist style and I felt that it fitted in with my sense of well being, in preparation for this particular meeting. If you had taken a photograph of me on Sunday and Monday, you would have seen the difference in hairstyle and appearance. On this particular Monday, I realised that I had succumbed to the unwritten rules syndrome. I began to reflect and found myself asking questions like what would happen if I went to work with my hair frizzy. What would people think? Would I be bothered about what they might say?

I came to the conclusion that I adapt my appearance to suit the external environment and society, including hearing the voice of my mother, "How could you go out looking like that, you have no shame, people aren't going to give you a job looking like that."

I cannot believe that in this day and age, and being a woman in my forties, I am pandering to society's expectations. I suppose the question is: in society, who is expecting certain behaviour and looks? Yes, we know about the media, the hair and beauty business, but, why can't I be satisfied with what God gave me in my natural state? Why do I have to shave the hair under my armpits and elsewhere? Are we doing this for ourselves or for others?

Can you blame the younger generation for following the media lead and dyeing their hair, wearing extensions and putting chemicals in their hair? Do they live through the dilemma of culture assimilation, or cultural survival? Seeing young black girls with blond straight hair saddens me as I wonder whether they are following fashion trends, attempting to look European or developing their own identity as young black people living in England.

This journey of life around hair has, with hindsight, highlighted the above issues, in one form or another, of wanting to conform, yet be different. Yes, I did the curly perms and relaxed thing, but after the birth of my daughter, 14 years ago, I have maintained a natural style, with no chemicals, and with occasional extensions, double twist or afro. My hair journey does not stop there, as I consider growing my hair into locs and what it means to me.

Everyday, there are unwritten rules, which consciously or unconsciously, dictate our behaviours and thoughts and probably once in a while we should pause and think: why do we deal with life the way we do.

AFRO CHILD

Suzanne Creaville

Ears scorched by the brusque, rapid brush movements causing bristles to scratch the tender lobes like a scorpion hot on its heels having dealt its deadly strike into its predator. Eyes like little slits; hoping, begging, and praying for the time to end, a time to break free from the clutches of the captor. Nerve ends pulsated into spasms, each brush stroke bruising the tender temples of my face into red steaks. Oh how hateful was this time each morning. Every day it was the same. When am I ever going to break free, "perhaps never" I dreaded. Shouts of protests and grimaces only brought more torture as mother seemed to become more impatient. Oh why I exclaimed at the young age of eight, did I not have "good hair"!

You know the kind of hair that was soft and wavy, the kind that you could brush in one fair swoop. *Girls' World* was my favourite doll, pulling out her hair extensions and combing and cutting was the favourite pastime. *Girls' World* had that soft, long European hair that was fun and manageable to play with. Instead, I was a brown skinned, high yellow, mulatto looking child with `nappy' afro hair. It was unheard of; forbidden, distasteful, troublesome, and rebellious according to all who encountered my hair.

"Tut tuts" and "Child, your hair is so coarse" was the usual chorus (except we were not singing any hymns) from the elders, peers and hairdressers, which was rapidly followed by agony: first the pulling that yanked me out of the chair as the comb tried its best to pass through the jungle and then rapidly followed by gasps of mental torture as I viewed the horror on their faces. This was not only a scorching of the temple but of the mind, as my fair skin and unruly hair was enough for me to hide inside as if in a cocoon waiting for the day it was safe to unfold, to crawl out and escape from the judgements with a new sense of self. Why did my mother have good, fine hair? Yet I, yes I, had the afro-kinky hair that was as resilient as coiled wire.

Neither grease, oil, shea butter, nor hot steam caps could soften that hair that shrunk to one third of its length after washing, like a spring needing to be stretched back into shape. It always reminded me of my baby picture with a chubby face and two inches of afro covering my scalp. Time passed but the inner turmoil did not.

Mama could no longer cope with the daily wrestling and so new methods were brought in to make life simpler. Endless years of straighteners, curly perms, tight plaits that literally pulled my scalp back and made my eyes slant, troubled the scalp like a raging red hot inferno. The chemicals leaving their destructive residue on my sensitive scalp was the price to be paid, not a cheap one at that! Plaits made me feel like a long haired queen and I no longer had to put the towel around my head, imagining the flowing, long hair like my childhood play.

Searching for a sense of freedom from the chemicals, I shaved my scalp and it was sheer joy to feel the breeze and not worry about combing. It was fun to go to the barbers and listen to the men in their daily chatter about cricket, football and boxing. People were curious about this new found look and there were a few petty remarks but on the whole it was a new found identity.

We do not always realise that the hair is a portrayal of self on which people make assumptions – it seemed to others that I was deemed as confident and non-conformist. Maybe, I was becoming that way but not purposely. With the change of hair, came the change of clothes as I could no longer wear baggy clothes and jogging pants, which made me appear boyish. Like the Queen of Sheba, I adorned myself in ethnic earrings and chokers, which symbolised my journey to freedom. The years passed and I started to twist my hair, the next logical step towards another journey, a time for change.

Age 33 and I always had a secret desire to locs my hair but worried about the social acceptability in the corporate world and my own insecurity, it had always liked the soft breeze of the wind murmuring its call. One day, I woke up and knew that it was time. The season had come for me to follow my spirit and locs my hair and paradoxically enough, I had the perfect hair type for locsing. So, my frizzy, coarse hair had found its home after all, a place where it could be at peace. By this time, natural afro hair of all types was now acceptable and black women were walking tall with dreadlocks, china bumps and short afros. There was no longer any need for me to be living out other people's expectations and now I stand with my head high, hair fanned out and love the sense of liberty it gives me in its thick, coiled spring.

Five years of long flowing dreadlocks down my back reminding me of my *Girls' World* and I was to face a new journey, a road map that I had not envisaged but one that resulted in the hair on my temples and in the middle of my head receding. Each morning, I noticed the straggly strands, the large gaps in my scalp that shone like a light reflector of the sun. Each morning, I prayed and swung my locks over my shoulders hoping for some miracle. I sought advice from one hairdresser to another, who only gave me some magic potion and told me to stop growing my locs.

Another said it was stress. Confused, anxious and reality shining its light on me on a Sunday morning, my hands reached out for the scissors (the big, household scissors by the way) and I snipped away until memories were short tufts. Each snip was difficult but the journey was one that needed to be taken. There are times when you just have to flow with the universe. Each strand I cut I placed into a bag and put it away in a drawer. I'm not sure why but maybe it will be something I pull out of my box of memories in my old age, or maybe I am putting the past to rest.

The first few days I admit were prolific. I had not only to face the world but also myself. The patch in the middle was obvious and I felt that people, well black people, were all looking at me. Walking past shops, the gym, where people had become accustomed to my locs, was a source of anxiety and fatigue.

Now, my hair is well rested and free from any tension and after a few months, the patch has become thicker. I am now enjoying the short crop and it has enabled me to become the funky diva that I am.

Black women are women of dignity and pride and some things are just taboo. We can talk about wanton lovers, the inequality in our jobs, the illnesses in our family and our children. We can support each other with food, laughter and love but we cannot ever admit that we have "coarse, hard, afro hair" or worse still, that we are facing hair loss. We dollop lashings of soft grease, texturise, jheri curl, weave. We loc, relax and press our hair in the hope that we can somehow never have to admit this to ourselves or others. I no longer look to be accepted. You have to accept yourself first before others will and I am secure in my being to be who I am and let others be who they are. So here I am, a brown-skinned girl proud to have my short, wiry afro hair that has a mind of its own.

No reasons, no explanations, no apologies needed.

I am what I am.

STILL A BIRD... BUT NOT A ROBIN

Yolande Deane

I remember playing "hairdressers" when I was in primary school; all the white girls would sit down on the playground bench to have their hair "done". Admittedly, other white girls would be the hairdressers too, but the white girls were *always* the clients in our shop because their hair was "easy." The second memory I have is waiting to go on stage for a Christmas play. All the white girls would get their hair brushed by the teaching assistants, they probably had no idea what to do with our plaited hair that did not move with the wind and felt like "cotton wool", as one of my white friend's dad said to me once, while I was at her house. I think from a young age as a black girl you come to see your natural hair as hard to deal with; it does not fall down your back and dangle there, waiting for you to flick it when it falls into your eyes.

Once I got to secondary school the next stage was to relax your hair....obviously, right? I mean why wouldn't you? It would make your life a whole lot easier, wouldn't it? However, I never quite got to that stage. My hair was hot combed two or three times. I had extensions put in twice but I never got round to the relaxing stage. It seemed to pass me by. I considered it when I was about 12 years old, but I think I was put off for life when a cousin of mine, who taught hairdressing, said that my hair would break off, I remember her giving some technical explanation, but the words "break off" just did not marry well with my adolescent vanity and I decided from that moment to "struggle on" with my hair. I think that comment from my cousin sent me on a hair journey that I never expected to go on. I thought *I'm stuck with it now.*

I will admit that I used to get angry with my hair. I just couldn't find a style for it; my hair seemed to rebel against every clip, scrunchy or hair band that I put in it. It would just spit it back at me with contempt as if it was saying "enough already!" But I prodded and I poked, and I blow-dried and I tried to gel – it wasn't having it. My hair was never going to be *wash and go,* I knew that, and my hair knew that, so we settled on wash and twist – that'll do I thought.

What amazes me is the amount of black women that have come up to me and asked me how do I get my hair to look like this; short curly twists, which is ironic to me because I don't "get" my hair to look like this, it *is* like this, and I often wonder if many black women have forgotten what afro hair is like due to years of straightening? I sometimes want to say "What do you mean how do I get my hair like this? It's your hair too" The next question they ask is "Do you think I can do my hair like yours?" I do not always know how to answer this question, because there is so much diversity among us as black people, that my natural hair for example, is completely different to my sister's despite the fact that we are both black. We are not a homogenous race; we seem to accept the diversity among others but not among ourselves. So the answer I suppose is "yes" you can do your hair like mine – if we happen to have the exact type of natural hair! If not, then your twists will look different – and that's okay too, because we don't have the same fingerprints now do we!

Since writing this piece I am even more aware of how closely identified I am with my natural hair. The thought of it being relaxed makes me think of a robin with its chest painted blue. It's no longer a robin, is it? It's still a bird, but not a robin.

THANK GOD I'M NATURAL!!!

Chris-Tia Donaldson

It was Saturday night and my place was *packed*!!! As *This Christmas* played loudly in the background, I could finally breathe a sigh of relief — knowing that for once everything was going exactly according to plan. This year, I decided to make things easy on myself. Instead of doing all of the cooking as usual, I simply picked up a shrimp platter, a veggie tray, and a few desserts from Costco's. All I had to do was take the teriyaki wings out of the oven. What could be simpler, right? Wrong!

No amount of preparation could have prepared me for what happened next. As I bent down and leaned my head towards the broiler, I could feel 475 degrees of intense heat sweep across my face and over my forehead, instantly transforming my wig's soft, flowing bangs into hard, melted plastic. It didn't take long for the unmistakable stench of burnt hair to permeate throughout my apartment and overpower the smell of everything, even the sweet aroma of my Glade Christmas-Cookie plug-ins! There I stood, melted plastic bangs glued to my shiny, sweaty forehead and my friends waiting in the very next room . . . still hungry.

Fortunately, not all was lost; I had a collection of 30 different wigs in my closet. Yes, I could look like Beyonce,

Ashanti, or any girl in a rap video for a mere $24.99. But with that terrific flexibility and variety, came a hefty price – paranoia. What if my wig was on crooked, or if, heaven forbid, a mighty gust of Chicago wind came and carried my precious hairpiece right down Michigan Avenue? Even worse was wearing a wig while dating! Let me tell you, while I had mastered the art of keeping men's hands out of *"my hair"*, it was a constant challenge (and emotionally quite stressful) to maintain my dirty little secret. Extensions are one thing to most men, but wearing a wig involved a whole new layer of deception that inevitably led to the *"Honey, there is something I have to tell you; this isn't my hair..."* conversation.

As I searched through my closet frantically looking for a suitable replacement, I sat down amidst the strewn clothes, shoes and hair pieces, and broke down in tears. Then, it hit me: I was happy wearing hair in every colour, texture, and length – but not my own. Seeing my charred wig lying on the dresser that night, forced me to come to grips with my kinky tresses. Like most black women, I had an unhealthy and sometimes negative perception of my hair. I knew I needed to let go and stop wearing a wig, but after two years of waking up every morning and putting one on, I couldn't stand the sight of myself without my synthetic tresses.

You see, I had recently decided to go natural, and although my hair was quite long, my hair looked dry and dull, like week-old cotton candy, because I had kept it covered for so long. After perming for over 20 years, I didn't know the first thing about caring for my natural texture. I had no clue what products or styling tools to use or how to work with the tight, spongy curls sitting atop my head. Learning to do my hair was like teaching myself Swahili. I simply didn't know where to begin. This episode forced me to come to the realization that me and my hair would be together until death do us part and was also the inspiration for my new book *Thank God I'm Natural: The Ultimate Guide to Caring for and Maintaining Natural Hair.*

Although going natural was a long, difficult and sometimes painful journey, it's one that I will never regret. My natural journey, which has been fraught with many difficult moments, has taught me many lessons (including not to retrieve appetizers from an oven while wearing synthetic hair) but most importantly, that we, as black women, must learn to love our hair, embrace our unique differences and no longer be ashamed of who we truly are. Today, I love my hair more than ever before and have just as many styling options, if not more (minus the paranoia) as when I was wearing a wig. While it has taken me close to 25 years to accept my kinky mane for what it is, I can now finally say, THANK GOD I'M NATURAL!

COILED JOURNEY

Rachelle Hull

In the beginning

My sister, cousins and I were on a mission as we scrambled through the chest of drawers, pulling out all kinds of jumpers: brown ones, red ones, long-sleeved and cropped ones. We laid them out on the bed, mulling over the possibilities. I picked the brown jumper, Chantelle chose a red one, my sister always went for the black cropped and Sabrina was left with the yellow sleeveless. All realistic colours. As we stood in front of the wardrobe mirror, we placed our selected jumpers on our heads, tweaking and pulling until the coils were covered. Satisfied, we continued to play.

For most of our childhood, my sister and I wore our hair in braid extensions. I don't believe my mum had an issue with natural hair; she (like a lot of black women) just didn't know how to take care of it. She had never been taught how to cane row and her plaiting skills needed work.

At age 14, I didn't like my hair. Having eczema on my scalp when I was a year old caused my hair to fall out and the wear and tear from years of braids left me with fine, short, kinky hair. Though I vowed never to relax my hair, two years later I made the decision to do just that. By this time my mum's hair was already relaxed; my sister's too. Initially I had a bob cut, eventually getting the Halle Berry crop. I loved my hair (as did my boyfriend at the time) and felt good. But bi-weekly trips to the salon, not forgetting a touch up every 3-4 months, was beginning to take its toll. Not just on my pocket, but how I felt about myself. I began to dread the long days spent amongst burning hair, burning scalps, spritz and spray cans; among women with long faces, flicking through magazines featuring shiny new (always straight) hairstyles. The women smiling from those glossy pages looked like me, but I no longer felt connected to what they were trying to sell.

Around the same time as my discomforts with my hair choices, I began to frequent internet forums, setup for (and by) the global black community. It was a place of solace, for us to get away from the mainstream and air our grievances, joys and beliefs. It was not a utopia. Like we already know, black people are not homogeneous but it was 'home' in many ways. I began to learn about the history of us (Africans) outside of a European perspective, discovering titles of books, authors and historical figures I had never heard of before and was really challenged by some views and opinions. I began to do my own reading, in between college, friends and 'getting my hair done'. I cannot pinpoint the exact moment I decided to stop relaxing my hair, but I remember it being in 2003. Only four years after my first relaxer.

In the middle

I grew my hair out using braids. I wasn't up for doing 'the big chop', not because I thought it was ugly, but because I didn't think it was a style that suited me. It took about 12-18 months before I was ready to unleash the 'fro. It wasn't very big (my hair has always taken its time to grow), but it was completely natural. The next few years were a battle. Not only did I have to learn how to take care of my hair (funny seeing as I was born with it), but I also had to readjust my thoughts on what my hair was *supposed* to look like. My feelings towards my hair would fluctuate between love at one end of the scale and dislike at the other. Back in 2004/2005 there weren't many natural hair salons or products for natural hair (if you had locs you were ok). The main issue was teaching myself how to plait, twist and cane row well (still haven't mastered the latter!) and also how to wear these styles. Magazine pictures ranged from Beyonce's goldilocks, to Erykah Badu's full on wig, to Mel B's bi-racial curls. Neither of these helped, but thank goodness for the internet! After a few years of struggle, annoyance and fleeting thoughts of going back to the 'creamy crack', I'm in a position where I am happy and comfortable with my hair. Obviously there are days when it gets on my nerves, but it's a healthy annoyance and not from the feeling that I and my hair are lacking something. Making sure I did my own hair (instead of giving up, resorting to braids or hunting down a salon) has helped me to grow *with* my hair.

In the now

My four year old niece is surrounded by women who love their natural hair (my mum now has locs and my sister's hair is natural) and has a range of books containing pictures of people that look like her. However, she does not live in a bubble and we have to combat her questions and comments that indicate the cycle is starting all over again; that indicate this is an issue bigger than simply choosing between *Dark n Lovely* or *Nubian Natural* products.

I sometimes find myself asking the question: what is the difference between relaxing one's hair and skin bleaching? For many this is like comparing apples and oranges but I still wonder, when both set out to alter the state of something and both use harsh chemicals to do it. So what is the difference? As far as I can see one is (more or less) acceptable while the other is not and one leaves results you can work with, whilst the other does not.

Many black women across the globe would argue to the death that relaxing one's hair is purely a choice. I believe it's much deeper than that. History, in many instances, plays a part in so many choices made today; from the politics of our countries, to the politics of our hair. I'm not writing to tell black women they shouldn't relax their hair, but only to quit taking this issue out of the historical context in which it belongs.

HAIR WARS: GROWING UP FRIZZY IN THE 1970s

Fiona Joseph

My sisters and I grew up in Birmingham, born to a mother from the city and a father who'd made his passage across the Atlantic, all the way from St. Kitts.

The romance between my parents seeded and then flowered at church. In my imagination I can see my dad's eyes meeting hers, while she clung to the altar rail and sipped wine delicately from a silver chalice... But if God had blessed their union, it was far from a given that 1960s' society would follow suit.

When my mum – then 19 years old and white – announced her intention to marry my dad – aged 28 and black – there were ructions. She was made to resign from her secretarial job in a solicitor's office. The senior partner sadly shook his head at her foolishness and predicted a life of doom and disaster for any *half-breed* child brought into the world. (Surely she must realise, he said, that such a child's career options would be limited to drug dealing or prostitution!). Mum fought back, told him what he could do with his job and stomped out.

Little did she know that dealing with the narrow-minded doomsayers would be a cinch compared to the battles she'd face with her sister-in-laws. As soon as my sisters and I were born, my mum and the aunties on my dad's side were locked in fierce combat – over how to style our mixed race hair.

For convenience, Mum kept our hair cropped short, in one-inch afros, and when I flick through childhood photographs I find myself both laughing and cringing at the way my sisters and I stood side by side looking like exhibits in a topiary garden. My aunties were aghast.

'For the love of god, plait it,' Auntie Carmen implored.

'Stop cuttin' it,' Auntie Agatha would add, eyes cast heavenwards in sheer despair. 'Let the poor children get some length an' their hair'll grow into long soft waves before you can say *Shirley Bassey*.'

But no one was going to tell my mum what to do. She took her position and was prepared to defend it, even if she was a lone soldier at a deserted gatepost.

'Look nuh! You cut them childs' hair *again*!' Auntie Carmen would beckon us over to stand next to her enormous bosom while she inspected the damage. She'd rub our heads with the flat of her hand like she was fluffing up the pile on a carpet, and then suck her teeth in disgust. She'd dig her fingers around in the frizz, and declare, 'You could hide a marble in that bush and not find it for days.'

I don't recall being upset by my aunties' comments. Perhaps I inherited my mum's defiant spirit, because I loved it when she cut my hair. The ritual began on a Sunday evening after bath-time. First, I'd stand on the settee in the living room to get the mirror down, always checking first that dad was elsewhere (feet on the furniture being a hanging offence in our house). Even today, I remember that mirror with its bronze-coloured leaves and curls, and how it took all my strength to lug it into the kitchen. Meanwhile, mum had got the dressmaking scissors from her sewing box and, with a towel draped over my shoulders, we'd be ready for our game of hair salons. I'd sit at the table, holding the mirror steady in front of me, until my arms ached and wobbled and I'd have to rest the mirror on my lap. As mum hacked away, spread out pages from *News of the World* would catch the clumps of almost-black coils.

'Stop playing with it – it gets everywhere,' she always said. But I'd still squeeze it into a pile and feel the lovely bounce of it. Cutting our hair was a very inaccurate operation – no rules, no technique, certainly no conditioner or oils – just chop and hope for the best. Mum was resigned to it: 'Your hair always does its own thing anyway.'

For most of our childhood, mum remained the victor in the war of the hairstyles. However, she did concede some ground to Auntie Agatha when her eldest son, our cousin, got married. Mum announced she was going to set our hair for the wedding.

'Can I get the mirror down?' I said. This was something new and therefore exciting. We had to sit for hours while mum stretched and coaxed our uncooperative hair around the rollers. That night we had to sleep in them.

The trouble my mum went to must have worn her out because she pleaded exhaustion and packed us off with my dad to our auntie's house.

Auntie Agatha opened the door, took one look at the rock hard rolls on our heads and declared, 'Well, bless the lord!' (For years I thought it was the *lard* she worshipped.) She bundled us through the hallway like we were fugitives, up the narrow staircase and into her bedroom, where she took a paddle brush to our hair. I've never forgotten the eye-watering pain of having our curls, cemented in with *Elnette* lacquer, tugged out. All my mum's efforts lay in ruins, annihilated. We wanted to stand up for her, we really did. I looked to dad for support but he, the abstainer from the conflict, just shrugged as if to say, 'just do what your auntie says'.

In the wedding photos we look as if we're wearing birds' nests on our heads.

The following summer, our cousin Mavis came to stay. Mavis was Auntie Agatha's 12 year-old daughter and it was arranged that she would have my bed while I bunked in with my sister. After mum had tucked us all up, Mavis reached in her bag and pulled out a rectangular piece of purple silk. I watched through one eye as she stuffed the pillow into the fabric before settling down to sleep with a smile on her face. In the morning the silk pillow case had gone and I wondered if I'd dreamt it until the following night when she repeated the ritual.

I couldn't resist asking, 'Why are you doing that?'

'It's to stop my hair from snagging.' Mavis wore her hair braided close to her scalp but that night she loosened it to show me; it was soft and wavy beneath my fingertips, rippling past her shoulders like a princess in a fairytale. For the first time I felt a flicker of doubt, a questioning. *Why didn't my hair look like that?*

This was July 1976 and there hadn't been a drop of rain for weeks. For three nights running the conversation between mum and cousin had gone like this.

'We really ought to wash your hair, Mavis. It's been so hot and sticky.'

'It's fine auntie, honestly'. But mum won the battle in the end.

'I'm not having her going back to your sister's with dirty hair,' she said to my dad.

Mum barred me from our tiny bathroom but I could picture Mavis bent forward over the sink while mum lathered her hair with *Vosene* medicated shampoo and then rinsed it in a basinful of fresh water, Mavis's tresses swimming in the water like mermaid's tails.

Minutes passed slowly and then mum poked her head round the bathroom door and saw me sitting on the landing.

'Get your dad,' she hissed. I asked why. 'Just get your dad.' He was on the back step with the radio pressed to his ear trying to catch the test match.

I followed him up the stairs just in time to see Mavis coming out with a towel around her head and mum behind her with a face like she'd been watching a horror film. Mum and dad disappeared into their bedroom and slammed the door shut.

I smiled at Mavis. The bits of hair that escaped from the towel looked all frizzy and matted, like fraying black rope. I just had time to wonder what had happened to her silken locks before her face crumpled and she ran off into my bedroom, leaving me free to eavesdrop.

'What on earth am I going to do?' my mum was saying.

'You got to fix she hair before she go back.' Typical dad, always stating the obvious.

'But it's shrunk to half its size. I can't even get the comb through it.'

There was only one thing for it. Dad plonked Mavis on the back of his Suzuki and they sped off to Auntie Carmen's. We waited two hours for them to return. I can still remember the coconut smell as Mavis walked back through the door, her eyes all red from crying, and her hair 'fixed' once more in braids that glistened, even in the dying light. My dad followed, his face a volcano, because he'd missed the cricket.

And on my mum's lips I remember a tiny smile, certainly one of relief that the crisis was over. But I swear there was a sliver of gratification too in her expression, a sense of triumph at a score having being settled. Nothing so obvious as a *deliberate* revenge on Auntie Agatha for ruining our wedding hair, but then again I wonder.

OUR CROWNING GLORY

Valerie Mason-John

Women of African descent spend more money on their hair than any other race of woman in the world. Why? Because they don't have the time in the West to socialise as our parents and grandparents would have back in Africa or the Caribbean. Preparing our hair would have been an important part of the female community gathering together and catching up on important gossip. Why? Because our hair dries out in colder climates, as a result of a lack of sun to feed our follicles, making our hair harder to manage. Why? Because as much as we'd love to, we just can't go to bed with our hair unprocessed and wake up in the morning and flick or shake our hair.

My hair for the most part has been unprocessed, and although I walk around the house in the morning trying not to comb out the knots, if I left my home, people would think I was the local mad woman of Brixton. Of course in white areas I would most probably get away with it. Many white people don't seem to notice if our hair has been combed or uncombed, and can often admire the natty look. However, most black people would not be seen dead, let alone alive, with hair that hasn't been combed for several days, unless of course they've pruned it into dredloks.

When black women migrated to England in the fifties and sixties from the Caribbean and Africa, looking after our hair was a problem. The only products available were petroleum jelly, royal crown a sweet smelling *Vaseline* and *Brylcreem*. And let's not forget the hot comb on the paraffin heater that singed our hair to a crisp. Today, when you walk in the black areas, there will be shop after shop carrying all sorts of products for our hair. Organic, vegetarian and chemical creams all vying for our attention. Within a half mile radius of Brixton, I have counted over ten hairdressers for black women, and they are all active social hubs of the community.

Most of my mother's generation living in England would have worn wigs as they had no time to sort out their hair, while having to take care of the children as well as going out to work. The seventies gave birth to more straightening products imported from the US. We could relax and perm our hair.

In the eighties, our hair became even more fashionable. The British media claimed that "Bo Derek invented the style of extensions and braids hanging with beads," funny that. Just like how some people claim that Madonna invented the form of dance called *Vogue*. However, we did see more shops opening and catering for black hair. Up until then, there was only really the black barber, who cut afros and shaved beards. We also began to see more products swamping the market for black hair; somebody had finally worked out that black women spend money on their hair.

While processed and permed hair was becoming a familiar feature for black women to don, the complete opposite of not combing the hair was emerging as a fashion, known as dredloks. Dredloks have been part of the history of every spiritual system. In Hinduism and Christianity, there are references to locked hair being a symbol of a person moving closer to God, a mark of spiritual status. In some African countries, they were seen as a mark of mourning. And In 1930, when the Emperor of Ethiopia, Ras Tafari, was forced into exile, the guerrilla warriors swore not to comb their hair until he was reinstated; hence their association to Rastafarianism.

Dredloks were brought into the British mainstream by the late reggae artist Bob Marley; his hairstyle initiated international interest. Dredloks became a fashion statement in the mid to late eighties and part of ethnic pride. However, because of their association to the Rastafarian religion, and Christians deeming the hairstyle as disgusting and frightening, there has been a stigma; hence the Christians gave the name 'Dread'. Dread being a derogative term, many Rastafarians reclaimed this term, by replacing dread with dred; hence the more popular spelling of their hair is dredloks.

Back in some Caribbean islands, school children would be heckled for sporting dreds, and some adults branded Rastafarians as thieves. This attitude followed us to England. Some black people ostracised you because they associated dredloks with trouble and being dirty. In the eighties, Rastafarians experienced a lot of police harassment, which didn't help the negative views about dreds during this period.

Then there are those of us who managed to break the mould. In the eighties we saw black women growing dreds and not putting it under a wrap. This was a cardinal sin to the Rastafarian religion, as a woman's hair must be covered at all times. Like the Muslim woman she should adhere to simplicity and modesty. I remember being in supermarkets and receiving long lectures from Rastafarian men telling me how my hair should be covered so I remained pure. This attitude has relaxed in the past twenty years. Now, the funky dred has become popular among our black brothers. The side of the head shaved, with dreds on top, designer dreds for aesthetics and image.

Dreds were also a revolution for black women whose hair didn't seem to grow, often if uncombed and locked her hair would grow as never before. In the 21st century black women have jazzed up the dredlok style to the extent that an employer would find her acceptable to employ, unlike in the eighties and nineties, when some corporate banks and offices refused to employ us if we had a head full of dreds. Unlike our black brothers, who still face stigma. Dreds for black women have become so fashionable, that many black women have temporary dreds twisted and woven in with artificial hair.

In the nineties, black women shaved their hair and became bald. It was a scary fashion for some black people to cope with. This was sacrilege – how could we do such a thing – bare our African features to all and sundry without any hair to hide behind? But the world had to admit that black women with bald heads did look beautiful. And then we bleached our hair with peroxide in the mid-nineties, which fucked up our hair, made it brittle and at worst it fell out in clumps. Some of us became Afrekeke; adopted some traditional African clothing styles, jewellery and hair dos. We learnt from the women of Ghana, Nigeria and other African countries how to tie a head scarf in beautiful and elaborate ways. But how radical were we? Black women have donned bald heads, blonde heads, dred heads and worn spectacular head wraps for centuries.

If you look at all the famous black women in the world, how many of them have natural unprocessed hair? Dear old Whoopee Goldberg and Grace Jones. And the media does not define them as beautiful. Now Naomi Campbell, Iman, Halle Berry, and many more, all have processed hair and are beautiful, so says the media.

In the UK we have Moira Stewart, the face of the national news for many years, Diane Abbott, the black female face of politics, Tricia Goddard, the face of chat show TV. But, don't be fooled, they all spend hundreds of pounds on their hair. Why? Because they are too busy to worry about their hair before they go to bed, and get up in the morning. Why? Because they are sensible. Well it's an opinion. Those of us who have managed to keep our hair unprocessed; untamed, uncensored, uncooked, are the true heroines. Joan Armatrading has been a true champion of the Afro. She's braved it through the seventies right up to today.

Hallelujah to Baroness Valerie Amos, for sporting the perfect unprocessed natural hair style; a short afro with shaved sides so she can sleep well and not have to worry about it all being squashed by the way she sleeps on her pillow.

It would be all too easy to say that black women wear extensions so they can be part of the *Barbie* revolution. It's more complex than that. But there is an argument for why our natural hair and canerow or braided hair doesn't make the fashion columns. Maybe more of us need to be brave and sport our natural hair, rather than spending hundreds of pounds to get the perfect Naomi Campbell look.

There are many stories told of a black woman's hair. Even today in countries like Surinam, hair is still a form of language, and a form of courtship. Each style is symbolic of a woman's marital status. A particular style or a way a head scarf is tied will inform a man that a woman is available. So you see the story of black hair could fill the British Museum, the Victoria and Albert Museum and the Tate Modern and that doesn't include black men. Speak to any black woman and she'll tell you a story or two about her hair.

BEAUTY MARKS AND BATTLE SCARS

Mesha Mcneil

Whoever penned the mantra 'Beauty is Pain' was probably the most insightful person of their generation. When it comes to a black girl and her hair, boy does she suffer? I've experimented with many different hairstyles and they all came with their tears.

It seems like a lot of women could do with that carefree attitude we had when we were children. When it came to my hair as a child, I could not give a damn. My mum always sorted me out however and wrapped pretty ribbons around my bunched afro puffs. When it came to my appearances as a kid I was not spoilt or overly self aware. I had better things to worry about such as climbing trees and forming a basis for my nostalgia like a kid should be doing.

It was every Sunday night where my platonic relationship with my hair took a turn for the worse. My mum would make it her mission to pass a comb through my thick head of hair. It would have been easier for my mum to straighten the branches of a bramble bush. Readers with kids might side with my mum and say I was over dramatic. "Stop crying or I'll give you something to cry about!" was my mum's Sunday night catchphrase. I'm pretty sure my grandma used to the say the same thing when my mum was a young girl.

After the weekly turmoil, we both got sick of the crying. My mum suggested extension braids; low maintenance, no trauma, everyone's a winner right? Wearing my new shoulder length braids, I walked past a friend in the hallway. She was a Sri Lankan girl with long raven hair. She gasped, mouth wide open and said 'Mesha, you look like a movie star.' That kind of positive reinforcement was enough for me to love my fancy new hairdo. The pretence of glamour shortly left my nine year old self when a reaction to the synthetic hair left me with psoriasis of the scalp. My entire head was as white as cigarette ash. Not to mention anyone that manages to get a child to sit still for three hours straight deserves a public holiday named after them.

After the distress caused to my scalp by combs and psoriasis, it looked like things could not get much worse. That was until I reached my adolescent years and I discovered the black woman's kryptonite – hair relaxer. There is something attractive to a teenage black girl about forcing your hair straight with corrosive chemicals applied near your brain. With no surprise the hair relaxer stunted the growth of my hair and aggravated my psoriasis, which would have disappeared if I had never placed chemicals on my hair. I wore relaxer throughout high school despite the trouble it caused my hair and scalp, which I protected with numerous treatments and potions.

After leaving high school, I decided enough was enough and I cut out the relaxer from my hair. I went full circle and started wearing my hair the way nature intended. I could wear my hair in an afro whilst my white and Asian friends could not. I needed to embrace that. There may be a lack of women with afros in the media but when I go out in London with my hair natural, my confidence to ignore what is acceptable certainly draws admirers.

I currently alternate between my natural hair and a low maintenance weave depending on my mood. I'm 20 years old; I'm allowed to be fickle about my image. Until my natural hair has recovered from the past damage I've imposed onto it, I will be protecting it underneath a hair weave. The current natural hair/hair weave combo is a sensible choice for me and allows me to feel beautiful without the painful baggage. Though I have to admit, a past experience with a badly applied weave must have made mine and everyone else's eyes sore.

"YOUR HAIR IS YOUR BEAUTY"

Pauline Walker

'Your hair is your beauty, why you cut off your beauty?' so said my mother when I turned 33 years old and she was 70.

My mum was Jamaican; she was half black (her mother) and half Indian (her father). Her scalp never needed to be greased up but she did it because that's what her mother and aunts did. I could tell mum was a bit annoyed at the quality of hair I'd inherited. She would pull apart the tight curls on my head and with her forefinger, paste the hair pomade onto my scalp. She would complain that the hair was real 'Negro' hair; why couldn't my hair be soft and pliable like my sister, Marcia's.

Marcia's delightful hair could be easily parted. She didn't cry when her hair was pulled taut and the comb began its backward journey. First the ends were teased, and then the comb went in mid-shaft. Finally, the teeth of the comb went in close to the scalp and Marcia's hair would slip through, tangle-free. Me, I would be alright when the ends were teased, but I'd start to tense up when the comb was chopped into the hair mid-shaft. By the time the comb was at the scalp I was crying.

'Keep your head straight,' mum would instruct me as

I twisted my neck and contorted my body, trying to minimize the inevitable pain by pulling the hair out of her hands. By the time she finished, my scalp would be tingling and the plaits were pulled so tight that I thought my head would explode when I lay down on my pillow.

Marcia's hair would never stay plaited. The curls refused to be tamed. An hour after plaiting, the ends would start to uncurl and the loose curls would be free. There were plenty of grips and elastic bands in Marcia's head. My plaits were obedient; they stayed where they were placed.

By the time I was 18, I decided to straighten my hair. So long as I wore it plain at church and didn't encourage the devil with a decadent style, mum was ok with that; she could see the advantage of easier combing. The pastor's daughter was the only young woman who didn't rush to the salon. She wasn't allowed, but she was canny – the bible didn't say anything about pressing one's hair with a hot comb.

Even though I straightened my hair, I was never adventurous with it. I never bleached it like my friends wanted me to and I never went for a Halle Berry short cut. It was always a boring ponytail with changeable scrunchies. However, in my late twenties I was forced to face the fate of my family – early on-set grey hair. I hated it so I started dyeing my hair black. I thought that no-one would go out with a woman in her twenties with grey hair. By the time I turned 30, I was getting tired of straightening my hair and the boring ponytail rut that I'd fallen into. I'd look at younger black women who had no compunction or fears about cutting their hair into any style, adding weave and colouring or bleaching.

When I had first started straightening my hair mum said, 'You must not cut it, only men have short hair, a woman's hair is her beauty.' I took that to heart; my hands would start to feel clammy and my heart would begin to palpitate when my hairdresser brandished her scissors, 'Do you want it trim?' she would ask. I would say 'No' and she'd reply, 'You have to trim it, to get rid of the split ends,' and she'd snip away. I would squirm in my chair like I did when mum used to comb my hair. I was determined to keep my hair as long as possible; it used to fall just below my shoulders. I was often accused of having a weave – it really couldn't be that long naturally, could it?

But I was getting fed up with the burnt patches on my scalp every time the hair was straightened and with asking my friend to home-dye it every two weeks to save on salon prices to stop the dreaded grey from peaking through. That was the problem with hair, the roots kept growing. I made a decision to stop dyeing my hair when I was 40. I thought that was a long way off.

When I was 33, I was braver. I went to the salon and asked them to cut my hair off. I started at number three and now I have a number one and a half. My mum was disconcerted when I turned up at her seventieth birthday celebrations. I looked too much like my brother Andy: 'Why you cut off your beauty?' she asked sadly.

When I was 40, I did stop dyeing my hair and let the grey do its thing. It wasn't easy at first, to reconcile my inner self with how I looked. I stood in front of the mirror and made myself confront the complete grey picture. I looked slightly older with it but my smile was still the same, I was still the same person. If people didn't like it, that was their problem. Some black women thought that I should have continued to play the vanity game and they told me so. I remember once at a friend's party, a black man asking me why my hair was the way it was. I have also had more positive reactions than negative since my short, grey hair came into being. Black and white women have approached me in the street to say they love my hair style. I remember my Aunt Lucille saying to my mum at her seventieth birthday dinner: 'It's ok. It's just a phase she's going through. She'll grow it back.'

I haven't and I'm 43 now. I think "Your hair is your beauty" was a repressive and limiting concept for me. It seems like we've always lived in a society where women are primarily defined by how they look but I don't care anymore. When I see my reflection in the mirror, I know my hair personifies certain aspects of my personality like being neat, tidy and disciplined. I also think it shows someone who is a risk-taker, someone who is willing to transgress and challenge what my mother's generation defined as beauty.

My hair is my beauty. It can also be whatever I want it to be. Ultimately, it's an expression of what's in my heart and that can change over time as my hair choices have.

NATURA POLITICA

Yvonne Witter

My hair story is one which is as eclectic as my life. I tell myself that my hair is the most beautiful feature of me. It's fantastically black, shiny, strong, thick and long, when I allow it to grow.

My earliest memory of the hot comb is that it was used for special occasions, like when I was flower girl at weddings in the sixties. I had to sit still and endure the heat from the comb, and the melting grease on my skull. Ouch. Then came the late seventies, and with it the dreaded 'cream'. The process always burnt and left scabs on my head, and for years left a scar on my forehead. I wonder whilst writing this, if these early experiences have affected my 'desire for beautification'. I have always viewed visits to the beautician with some trepidation.

Over the years, as I had my hair 'creamed', I never got used to sleeping with a head full of hard plastic rollers, plus these rollers are not even good for our hair as the hair gets wrapped in the sponge and breaks. 'Beauty' seems to be firmly established in my mind as a 'painful experience' and one which I need not endure. I can assuredly say that my early experiences have coloured my view of beautification as an 'unnecessary painful experience'.

In the seventies, came liberation thanks to my teenage rebellious phase. I could no longer be taken to the hairdressers every fortnight for that arduous experience. In my teens I had control over my hair. I sported an afro and defied anyone to predict my next hairstyles. Short fro, long fro, almost bald-headed fro. I had Angela Davies, the American civil rights activist and Black Panther member as a reference point. As I embraced the political revolution and democratic socialism of the late seventies and early eighties, I also tentatively embraced Rastafari. Bob Marley's *WAR* lyrics spoke to me and for a brief spell, I wore a red, green, and gold 'tam' knitted woolly hat but feeling confined by the religious dogma, I decided it was not for me. As I learnt about Garveyism and read Malcolm X's autobiography, I started to question the need for a perm and admired my beautiful African self. Yet I was also deeply fearful that this African self would be rejected by the outside world so I compromised and wore extension plaits, which I hated – before moving onto perms and chemically straitening my hair. I cut my hair short, I wore jheri curls; not quite straight and not natural either. The main problem was that I did not know hot to 'manage' my natural hair. I could barely plait it, so I always returned to what seemed the 'easiest' option.

It was the early eighties and it was in New York where I saw on a black t-shirt worn by an African-American male, written in large white letters 'Hands off African plaits – Who's Bo Derek anyway?' I never forgot the image. I had full control over my hair; there was no need to be rebellious. There was an underlying conscious need to feel comfortable in my own skin.

I searched for who I was in the world and found that an 'African in the Diaspora', regardless of a Caribbean heritage was and still is my true self. When I visited the spiritual home of Ghana in 1994, I was wearing locks. I was a mature student then and thought about a career in the arts, which I felt would allow me the 'freedom' to wear my hair, in what was considered 'unconventional styles'. After leaving University, I started to feel uncomfortable with the 'disapproving looks' from middle-aged black women I walked past on the street. This experience caused a nagging feeling that 'work' would be difficult with my natural hair also. It wasn't. I worked in Community Development within a local authority. Still, I cut the locks but sported a natural look.

I still struggled with my self perception, and career progression. I really did not mind my hair natural, but I was more concerned with what other people would think. I wore straight-haired wigs to work, covering my natural hair. Internally, I was intensely uncomfortable with the squeals of delight from my white colleagues on how 'fantastic' my 'hair' was. Did I need to wear a wig to feel accepted? NO. I needed to accept myself. So what, my colleagues preferred 'my hair' when assimilated as their own; it made sense. What did not make sense was my inner turmoil.

Eventually, I dropped the wig and the weave wearing. A temp joined our office who had her long tresses neatly managed; everything about her was neat. That was my turning point. To this day I think it is really important to acknowledge sisters who are courageous to go natural and applaud young women who are not processing their hair. We all need the support and encouragement as we are in the minority and often chided by friends and relatives.

In 2003, I established my own business and felt true freedom. I was now in control of my earnings. The growth of locticians like *Morris Roots* and hair grooming specialists in natural hair was a bonus. These salons were places of great comfort, reassuring and affirming in their service and dedication to keeping it all natural.

In late 2008, I hit a buffer on nearly all areas of life one lonely Friday night I cut my hair off, all of it. The reaction from people was mixed but most mourned the loss. I look back on that act as a form of self mutilation. Did I feel better after cutting it? I missed the sensation of running my fingers through my afro. But, the change, that immediate gratification, felt good. I needed a change in my life more than anything and my external circumstances were not moving fast enough. I learnt from that experience that it has been a pattern for me throughout my life – cutting off my hair in times of crisis. When I feel strong and centred, I wear my hair naturally with pride. When I feel derailed by the vagaries of love and life, the hair is cut.

Straightening is now completely out of the question, I would never consider it, nor would I wear a straight-haired wig. I would feel false, like a fraud. It just does not make any sense to me at all. Why do so many of us women of African origin want to wear other people's hair and synthetic hair? Why do we want to mutate our hair? I wish we loved ourselves more.

What is funny is the prejudice that endures about dreadlocks. It was interesting how some family members and friends commented favourably on my dramatic cut in 2008. However, I was not thrown by their comments; I now know what they were thinking when I had my dreadlocks. The difference for me is that I now know who I am and that I feel very comfortable.

Hair for me is personal and political. In June 2009, I started to grow my locks again. This time I am committed to having more control over the grooming of my hair and decreasing my dependence on salons. I am learning about natural products, applications and types of combs. I do not intend to cut my hair again except for styling. I intend from this day forward to truly love and appreciate my hair as a part of my natural beauty; something that I took for granted before.

PERSONAL ESSAYS: SKIN

*"Until people can look at themselves
in the mirror and say "My black is shine",
they will feel the need to change their skin colour
in order to be accepted, or feel beautiful."*

Belinda Otas *My Black is Shine!*
In *New African Woman* Autumn 2009

TO BLEACH OR NOT TO BLEACH?

Ellen Aaku

'Your soap will bleach my hands!' My four year old son goggled at me in such alarm; one would think I had asked him to eat my soap not wash his hands with it. His outburst was in the presence of six female members of a writers' group I had recently joined and was hosting for the first time. My guests had just entered my living-room and I was welcoming each one of them with an emphatic; *mwa! mwa!* cheek on cheek kiss when my son barged in. Although he was covered in white sand and had watermelon juice trickling down his tummy, his appearance before my guests didn't half embarrass me as did his disclosure about the ingredients of my soap.

My daughter, aged eight, old enough to realise her mother needed rescuing but obviously too young to be subtle, popped into the living-room, grabbed her brother by the arm and whipped him out. Before shutting the door she hissed, 'Mummy doesn't bleach!'

My face blazing, I hastily settled my guests and heard myself squeak, 'I've had spots since I was 13 and so I use a skin lightening soap to fade them.' As I spoke I presented both sides of my profile to the room and felt a rush of irritation at my foundation for flawlessly concealing my evidence.

As most embarrassing moments, it passed with an awkward silence quickly broken by an outburst of trivial conversation and inflated laughter, after which, the group settled into the writers' group business, as if my son had never happened. Although I passed around the tea and biscuits with a smile and made a hearty attempt at contributing to the discussion, I couldn't focus. My son's exposé had me feeling as if I had been caught cheating and I felt that everyone in the room thought the same of me.

My humiliation wasn't about betraying my roots; I've never had any qualms flaunting brown synthetic tresses that have no semblance to my natural kink. And had my son burst in and announced I wore fake eye lashes or that I dyed my hair I would have waved his words aside with a light hearted comment and let the moment pass. So what was it about being exposed as a bleacher that made me as defensive and secretive as an addict?

My earliest memories of skin bleaching creams are of an energetic neighbour who seemed to live in blue sponge hair-rollers and a pink nylon nightdress with a stained neckline. She lived her life sweeping, watering her vegetable patch or kneeling over a big metal basin filled with soap suds. As she invested so much time on domestic chores, one day I wondered aloud why she wore a dirty nightdress. My bemused mother explained that the neighbour's nightdress was not dirty but stained by skin lightening creams.

My mother went on to tell the story of how in her secondary school years she was sent off to boarding school stocked with jars of skin lightening creams purchased by her well-intentioned older sister. Those were the days when the general view was that one was either yellow-skinned and beautiful or black- skinned and ugly; my mother opted to remain in the latter category. And so she suffered the wrath of her older sister for stepping off the train at the end of each term with a black face. Apparently, my mother gave all the excuses she could to explain why her skin tone remained unchanged despite the regular supply of *Metamaphorsa,* because she didn't have the heart to tell the simple truth: her natural skin tone suited her just fine.

A few years after my mother had shared her views on skin lightening products, I travelled on a journey from Lusaka to Lubumbashi in the then Zaire. We drove in a sky blue VW Kombi with an aunt, my sister, cousins, suitcases, cans of powered milk, loaves of bread and dozens of boxes containing tubes of *Ambi Extra for Men* skin bleaching cream. Once we crossed the border into Zaire, my aunt retrieved a carton of *Ambi* from the back of the Kombi and nestled it in her lap as if it were a newborn baby. It wasn't long before we came to a big tree trunk lying across the road. We rolled to a halt and our Kombi was immediately surrounded by a dozen or so armed soldiers. With a serious look on his face, one of the soldiers wearing dark sunglasses and a thick gold chain around his neck, stepped up to my aunt's window. The other soldiers moved in close and stuck their faces against the windows, their rifles disconcertingly close. I didn't understand Swahili. However, from the tone of their voices I got the gist of the conversation between the soldier and my aunt, who happened to be a seasoned traveller on that route. The soldier pointed at the box in my aunt's lap and authoritatively asked a question. In a cajoling tone my aunt lifted the box flap slightly. Peering over the top of his sunglasses the soldier looked into the box and his expressionless face creased into a wide smile. He quickly reached for the box and shouted a command that snapped his men into action. The tree trunk was speedily hauled away from our path and we were sent on our way. The image of the soldier standing with a rifle slung over his shoulder, the carton box of *Ambi* skin lightening cream lodged in the nook of his arm and a grin on his face, stayed with me for years.

So up until then, skin lightening products were for housewives and jewellery-clad soldiers. Then I turned 13, and with the advent of my puberty came a bounty of black spots that could put a leopard to shame. Whilst my peers spent their pocket money on Babycham and vinyl records, I used all the kwacha I could get my hands on to purchase whichever product that promised to blitz my spots. In my desperate quest for clear skin, I slapped unorthodox remedies such as warm lemon juice, a paste of water and ashes and even toothpaste onto my face. I stopped short of snail slime because I didn't have the stomach to look at a snail let alone touch one.

Then I saw a TV advert for a skin toning cream. To the back drop of a disco hit and psychedelic lights, the advert showed a group of males in a nightclub swooning over a smooth, orange faced female with a toothpaste smile and an afro to die for. She breezed past everyone, hopped onto a bar stool and with a sip from a long stemmed glass, she swore that the only reason she had flawless skin was *Clear-tone* skin toning cream.

I bought into it.

Clear-tone didn't fade all my spots away as it pledged, but at least it faded them from black to dark brown. I had always been fairish, more toffee than chocolate. *Clear-tone* turned my black spots brown and the rest of my skin beige. At almost the same time I discovered *Clear-tone*, I happened upon liquid foundation for women of colour. And so once I had gotten over the teething stages of foundation stained collars and brown finger print smudges on everything I touched, I felt for the first time that I was winning the fight against my spots. That was how I started – lightening my spots – not bleaching.

You see, before my son's disclosure, despite using skin lightening products for years, I had never considered myself a bleacher. After all, I nudged and tittered with everyone else at the sight of an orange face on a black body.

Plus, I used safe over the counter products, not the banned skin lightening products some women used and ended up with purple patches of dead tissue on their cheeks. Even more significantly, I couldn't possibly be a bleacher, after all, hadn't my mother, who was of a time when skin bleaching was as enviable as owning a stiff under-petticoat and mastering the hand jive, shunned it?

I sincerely believed that because I didn't fit into what I considered to be the profile of a bleacher and because I used skin lightening products to clear my spots not lighten my skin, I wasn't bleaching. Hence my horror when in his innocence my son forced me to look in the mirror and face the facts.

The reality is that after 30 years of succumbing to the allure of the multitude of skin lightening creams on the market that promise to clear my skin, it's unlikely that I will wake up one day and miraculously find it in me to resist them. So perhaps instead of denying or justifying my vice, the way forward is to acknowledge it.

Here goes: My name is Ellen and I am a bleacher.

SKIN PERSPECTIVES

Natalie Ambersley

In the seventies, when my Jamaican father and English mother started dating, mixed race relationships were heavily frowned upon. Thankfully, by the time I came along in the early eighties the issues surrounding mixed relationships were starting to fade. The fact that certain people disapproved of my parents and their choice to bring 'mixed' children into the world was irrelevant. From an early age my parents taught me how to embrace both sides of my culture and be proud of who I am.

I grew up on an East London estate where skin colour was never really an issue and all races – black, white, Indian and Asian – mixed. My school was multicultural; everyone was friends with each other and I loved being a part of a close community. This feeling lasted until I was 14. My mum, believing I would get a better education, sent me to live with my grandmother in a suburban part of white Essex. It was at this point my skin colour started to play a huge part in my life. As I said goodbye to all my school friends and close-knit community I knew around the estate, little did I know my new school and area was predominantly white. There were over 600 students at this school with as little as ten percent being made up of another ethnic minority. It was very clear there was a strong racial divide when I was put in a class with 25 white students.

With all my new friends being white, I was quickly seen as the 'darker' one or the one with the 'caramel' skin, the one that could get away with not having to sunbathe, the one who had frizzy, uncontrollable hair, the one with a black dad. However, none of this was spoken with malice. Yet, the more I became aware of this, the more I was embarrassed by my black heritage. By the time I turned 15, I descended into an 'identity crisis'. I was embarrassed to have brown skin. I had become so accustomed to being amongst all my white friends that I started to wish I was white as well. They were all born at the same hospital, had gone to the same schools since they were kids and all looked like each other. I just wanted to be part of that, and not feel like the odd one out. At the time, I did not feel guilty about these feelings but when I look back I feel ashamed that the power was there to make me question who I was.

Luckily, those feelings were short lived. When I left school and experienced the 'real world', I found a new appreciation for my mixed race heritage and felt blessed that I was a part of two very different and enriched cultures. I was proud to have caramel coloured skin and tightly curled hair.

There have been many terms used to describe a mixed race person, for example, half caste, Brownie, half breed. All derogatory terms, but the worst term by far is 'confused' (about their identity). How can someone produced out of love be confused? I find it intriguing how people in society see me and often I think that the confusion comes from the wider society. Over recent years I have found black people see me as a mixed race or a 'light skinned' person, whilst white people see me as a black person. Generally, I feel that black people are more accepting of me as a mixed race person. They understand that even we, as mixed race people, go through issues surrounding the colour of our skin the same way they do. Like many, I have gone through times when the colour of my skin has left me feeling self conscious. Sometimes, when I walk into a bar and notice the majority of the crowd is white, I automatically feel a little self conscious, as though everyone is staring at my skin but never seeing me. Often, I start looking round for another person of colour, hoping to find shared solace in our skin similarities.

When people see me with my mum, do they automatically assume she is my mum? Do they think we can't be related because our skin colour isn't the same? Sometimes, I make a point of shouting "Mum" in a slightly higher tone, just so they look around confusingly and realise that 'the white lady' is in fact my mum. It seems my white mother's contribution to my life pales to insignificance because I do not have white skin.

As a child growing up, my dad would always talk to me about back home and what a beautiful country Jamaica was. He would always play the sounds of Bob Marley, Dennis Brown and Beres Hammond around the house before I even knew who Five Star, Mel and Kim and Bros were! All of this was a part of me understanding my identity, my colour and who I am.

After all the negativity, issues and perceptions surrounding skin colour, the reality is this: if we were to be stripped of our skin, we would all look the same, a walking pile of bones. So why does skin determine how we see each other, and how you see me?

A DAUGHTER TAKES A MOTHER ON A JOURNEY BACK TO HERSELF

Margaret Auguste

My daughter, aged six, sat on my lap and said to me, "Mummy why do you say you are black like us when really you are white?" I stared at her speechless as I collected what parenting skills I had left to explain to her that even though I have lighter skin than hers, I am still a black person just like her. She looked at me clearly unconvinced, while other comments ensued like, "Why is your hair brown when mine is black?" and "Didn't I think her hair colour was pretty?"

I had always perceived that any questions or issues surrounding skin colour or racial identity would come from society; an external source – an innocent but insensitive comment from another child, at school or on the playground. I never thought or prepared for the possibility that the source of any confusion or doubt regarding this issue could also come from me.

Immediately, forgotten memories of my childhood resurfaced. As a black woman who grew up in the eighties in small town America where I was the only black child in my kindergarten class, the issue of skin colour had been for a time, first and foremost in my life. Growing up as a light brown skinned black girl I had mixed messages about skin colour. "Black was Beautiful" I was told, but that expression caused some eye rolling amongst some of my older relatives who still believed that light skin was more desirable. "Black is Beautiful" also failed to resonate with most friends and acquaintances as I often found that amongst black and white people alike, I was too light for some and too dark for others.

However, as the years went by, American society seemed to really change in its perception of colour and beauty as I transformed with it, becoming sure of my place in this world. This year, incredibly, we elected Barack Obama, our first black president with mixed ethnicity and even better, a beautiful and accomplished dark skinned black first lady, Michelle Obama. In my mind the colour issue was over and as a busy adult I really didn't feel the sting of colour consciousness anymore or at least was too busy to notice it.

Nevertheless, I had vowed that if I ever had children that they, unlike me would never have doubts about this issue or have any negative experiences regarding skin colour. No matter what colour they were, they would feel proud and happy with themselves. I thought that I had successfully addressed this issue by providing diverse toys, dolls, books and movies and by even controlling our living situation by purposely moving to a the most racially and ethnically diverse suburban neighbourhood in New Jersey. The life I had created for my family, I concluded, was perfect, with no hint of racial tension or emphasis on skin colour and its possible negative connotation in our society. So why then, was my child making these disturbing statements?

My daughter's shocking words caused me to realize that maybe I was so prepared to address the expected, external factors that perhaps I was unprepared for the internal and the unexpected – my own children's startling observations about race and the doubts, fears and emotions that they stirred within me.

I decided that maybe I needed to re-examine my experiences by starting at the beginning. I became an instant parent with the curious experience of having four children in two years. I adopted my two oldest children and was blessed again, when approximately one and half years later I gave birth to fraternal twin boys.

When I first met my adoptive children, the African-American social worker hesitated before she introduced me by saying, "Now you realize these children are beautiful chocolate drop children," as if to warn me that they were dark skinned. Her reaction made me question myself. Did I give off a vibe because I have light skin that maybe I would be disappointed if they were not at least light brown skinned? She was also a "chocolate girl" herself and I wondered if she had been teased or devalued because of her dark skin and was maybe transferring these feelings onto the children. Should I have spoken these thoughts to her? Probably, so maybe it would have started an honest discussion but of course I said nothing and just gave her a small smile.

More colour issues were to follow with the birth of my twins who at birth they were as they say, "Light bright and almost white." Through the haze of my epidural my husband's eyes smiled at mine over his surgical mask as he held the babies and I knew just what he was thinking – *I bet all these white doctors and nurses are wondering where we got these white babies.* Our amusement continued throughout my hospital stay as new nurses and doctors saw my babies and their eyes widened. It continued after we took the babies home and our friends and relatives also voiced their opinions. "Are they going to stay that colour" asked my husband's co-worker as she held them on her lap at their christening. "They are too white" said my husband's disapproving Haitian Aunt, in her heavily accented Creole. "I hope they turn black like our family." She then offered to send to Haiti for a potion to speed their colour change along! I respectfully turned it down. My family of course was thrilled and triumphant; "they look like us" was the common refrain.

They did eventually get a "little more colour." One twin has very light vanilla skin with sandy, slightly kinky hair while the other one has brown skin and straight smooth black curls. We get even more of a laugh at people, both white and black, who do a double take when they see them together. They seem fascinated by the idea that twins can have different skin colours, oh my! When our entire family of six is out together we get even more looks but people seem to resolve it amongst themselves and I can almost hear their thoughts, *okay the older ones look dark like the husband and the little ones look like the mother.* In fact, I don't often have to imagine their thoughts because many people have made that exact comment or similar ones to my face – in front of my children.

I realised that my experiences were a mirror of her experiences and that what she really needed were not more black dolls and books but me. My authentic self being honestly presented to her so that she knows that the feelings she has are something we share as mother and daughter and as black women together. I dug deep within to find tools to be able to share my experiences with my daughter.

I decided to begin by drawing upon generations of experiences. My daughter loves to look at our antique family pictures because she loves the long old fashioned dresses, shoes and family stories of days long ago. I told her a story that I had never shared with her before about my Great Grandmother. She had white skin and red hair and was often mistaken for a white person. When she would go out with her children she would often be offered a chance to sit in the white section of the train and the local movie theatre but she would always refuse and go to the, "Negro section" with her children and friends.

She was riveted to this story even though she had a hard time believing that black and white people were ever separated in such a crazy way and was totally perplexed by what a "Negro" was or even how to pronounce it. Nevertheless, she got the main idea family was family, no matter what anyone had to say about it.

Finally, being honest with my daughter allowed me to be honest with myself; she was beginning to start her own journey in forming her identity and perception of self, just as I did and am still in the process of doing. She was trying to determine her place in our family and in their world in a context that made sense to her and addressing and understanding the part that skin colour plays in that journey was an essential piece of that journey.

As African-Americans, skin is not just our physical representation. It regulates our body temperature, eliminates toxins and acts as a barrier and filter for our bodies. However, our physical relationship to our skin colour is not only external but both personal and intimate with our personal physical relationship being intertwined with an emotional and psychological component as well. Our myriad skin colours are a living testament to our history in this country. It took my daughter's questions to enable me to pick up on a journey I had long since mistakenly thought was behind me so that I could embrace my true self and help my daughter embrace hers.

BRIGHTER DAYS FOR AFRICAN BEAUTY

Amanda Epe

I look in the mirror and see a copper-bronze caramel complexion smiling back at me. I love my skin and all that it represents at this point in my life and I live in the present. However, I haven't always had this sentiment. My era of animosity goes back to my early childhood starting at primary school. All my classmates, except two black girls and a mixed race girl were white European girls. Along with one of the black girls, the mixed race girl eventually left the school, but during her stay, I envied her. I envied her skin; she looked more like them, and she could be them.

My skin exposed me during my childhood of animosity. My classmates would often question why I was black. When it came to birthday parties my invitations came with the stipulation: "My mum doesn't mind blacks." The good, the bad, and the ugly – the good was the beautiful brown girl, the bad was the xenophobia from a few ignorant children and the ugly was the discrimination felt from some adults at such a young age. When people say "It's because I'm black", I don't wonder, I know and I understand.

With a good dose of parental empowerment, my inner desire to emulate others quickly faded and I grew into my skin, but the trigger for these changes came with secondary school and meeting other children like me, with the same skin tone. The experience gave me more skin perspective. At primary school I knew I was a black child, but not a milk chocolate, chestnut, or honey skinned child; I knew nothing about complexion. We as a race, when it comes to black skin complexion, discriminate against ourselves, even further than white people. The so-called blue-black, dark skinned pupils became targets for bullying, or were we just kids and was that part of growing up to pick on people? Where did this notion arise that being dark-skinned is ugly for 11 year old children? Within the black community, we have segregated ourselves into complexion categories: light/red skin, fair, brown, dark, black, jet black; the darker the colour, the more problems.

One weekend I was shopping with my mother and we were spotted by school friends. I was confronted with the statement: "Surely your mum can't be African – she is so light." This is the perception of Afro-Caribbean Brits and white pupils alike. Africa equals darkness and darkness equals Africa. Back then black children were preoccupied with complexion. Today, we are obsessed and its representations threaten to further divide the collective black community

Conscious of beauty, at least what I thought to be beauty, I invested in mountains of jars, tubs and tubes of creams. I had oily skin, pimples, spots, blemishes, blackheads and scarred skin. I wished I had a darker complexion, paradoxically on seeing celebrities and black icons on TV; I also admired their skin, as they notably were lighter blacks. A popular topic amongst both my Afro-Caribbean and Asian friends was skin complexion. There was a consensus that fair skin was nearly always perceived to be more beautiful and desirable; the lighter, the whiter, the better. Whilst I was content with my complexion, fleetingly a guilty yearning would covet a complexion a shade lighter, but these guilty moments would manifest during employment. I worked in a company where black employees were the tip of the iceberg and I often wondered if, being a light-skinned Eurocentric-looking black woman, I would be treated more favourably.

In my experience, it seems like a western concept where being a minority in some areas, specifically education and/or the workplace, has a profound impact on the way we see and feel about our colour and complexion. I once believed our issues of colour emanated from being a black minority living amongst the white majority, but I was wrong. On my first journey to Nigeria, I was faced with damaging consequences of skin complexion, especially the preference for and desire to be light-skinned. Many women, all ready quite light in complexion, were burning their skin with bleach to become allegedly more beautiful, regardless of the risks. Beautiful dark-skinned women were berated and insulted, "so black, blackie, go scrub", while light-skinned children were the pride of families. I could not get my head around the ideologies and paradoxical statements in Nigeria, where they insist on holding their pre-imperialist culture and identity. Yet the very same people idolize and crave for light skin and 'whiter looking' women.

There are no masters, there are no house servants, no field slaves; black people have come a long way from the days of slavery. But we have continued to carry the burden of this complexion legacy and hierarchy that deems one complexion worthy over another. This is the black culture's equivalent of the Brahmin caste culture, but there is no need for it. And yet, where history has bred this mentality, the media has reinforced it, with mainstream black celebrities continuously being fair-skinned, we need to define our own aesthetics and appreciate the diversity in our complexions, both dark, fair and the shades in-between. All over the globe, beauty lies within the beholder. If in the continent we stop sucking our western mother's breast and craving all western themes, perhaps then there will be brighter days for African beauty.

For me, skin complexion has gone from institutional racism and xenophobia, black UK colour discrimination amongst ourselves, young women's beauty ideologies, to British private corporations' views on black skin. My skin is important to me, and I love my unique DNA. I was created and fashioned perfectly as we all are.

WHAT DOES YOUR DRESS SAY ABOUT YOU?

Donna-Marie Glashen

If your skin was a dress, what would it look like? I ask, because I have some food for thought. When I smoked and ate on the run, the texture of my skin was dry, loose and wrinkled like linen; it was various shades of faded chestnut brown with black poker dots – very similar to an army camouflage print – my dress screamed war.

Because of the disproportionately high instances of heart disease and diabetes amongst women of African descent, I believe they are faced with similar skin in the morning mirror as they get ready to take on a world, which demands that we multi-task, stretching the seams of our tailoring to its limits.

Walking in May Pen market, Jamaica, during my rehabilitation from the rat race in 2009, I watched many black and mixed race women soldiering about their daily business, wearing skins, which divulged stories of battles, pride, poverty, privileges and self-esteem, while others in the heat were figuratively wrapped in cloaks.

I have seen this scene played out in the markets of the UK, America, Africa and Asia too. Actually, wherever there is a large population of women, especially of colour, you will find those who leave their skins exposed to reveal its full glory and there will always be those who choose to wrap it in make-up and/or bleaching products. Not that I want to stand in judgment of those who wear cosmetics, but I personally had got to the point where I couldn't walk down the high street without donning my warrior mask and found this a problem. What had happened to my dream of being a natural goddess?

Well, as a woman of Afro-Caribbean descent, I had eaten a fair amount of greasy chicken and an assortment of fried, heavily salty food, which had taken a toll on my skin – I began to look as seasoned as the food I ate. I estimate that a fair amount of women of African descent have probably also suffered break-outs (of the spotty kind) like me, due to the fast paced, heartless city life they live.

Like many young, underpaid, independent women of colour trying to achieve their goals, I felt pressured to counteract the constant stereotypes of black women being lazy, aggressive and over-sexed and tried to maintain a lady-like appearance, whilst being forced to battle like a man, but without the fringe benefits. I started working at the age of 15 years old and by my early twenties I exhibited a workaholic mentality; clocking up long hours to make money and running my own business in tandem with feeling like a hypocrite. I was not doing as I told my mostly female clientele to do – love themselves. I was always fighting the run-down type of flu (founded in cold damp London) with pill remedies.

I had been to war and to hide it I immersed myself under a thick layer of muddy foundation, bronzer and powder, (too much on many occasions) which stripped my natural complexion of its youthfulness leaving a faded Cuban portrait, crackled on close inspection from bad oil paint. My Cuban ancestors would have been horrified. My only saving grace was my slim figure (a result of running around all day) disguising my unhealthy eating habits.

Two things did jolt me into action, firstly health issues; I developed a case of gastritis because my stomach lining had an allergic reaction to vitamin supplements I had been taking (another short-cut remedy for not eating enough fruit and vegetables) combined with a case of food poisoning after treating myself to some very sweet, spicy, greasy ribs. I was left ill for weeks and my stomach initially would not allow me to return to my former bad habits.

Secondly, a conversation regarding make-up sold to black women in America, where I was informed that they found foundations containing skin stripping chemicals. I was surprised, but not shocked as my own skin was patchy and faded after a year of using an American brand of foundation.

Luckily, my worth is not defined by the hue of my brown skin, but it does represent a means of expression and I did not want to appear to bleach and condone it as if I were ignorant of the connotations associated with its use. Other women may give the impression of not caring, wearing their bleached skins mimicking European complexions in the markets all over the world with pride, whilst covered in shiny black poker dots, but I believed I could do better.

Whilst it can be argued that cosmetic companies should have a responsibility to inform their customers of the stripping affects of the ingredients in their products, I did not want to wait for them to change in order to transform myself. I left my busy life style with only one note on my Face book profile – 'I need a new dress'.

Waving the white flag, I admitted defeat, and stopped being a soldier at war by going AWOL. A bomb shell, worn down by my own expectations in an image conscious society; I took my dress off the shop floor before it was put into the sales bin and dry cleaned it by quitting smoking, drinking and greasy foods.

Several months in the Caribbean rehabilitated my art

attack; I weaned my body off toxic substances like a junkie. My drug had always been to look after others and like many women of colour, it was a consequence from lacking a constant father figure who had blamed his absence on his many problems and because I could not solve his issues, I compensated by attempting to solve everybody else's. So for me, this was the first time I unselfishly loved myself, like I had unselfishly loved and cared for others.

I do wonder how many black and mixed race women have this opportunity. I'm sure many have un-pampered bodies that are abused far worst than my own and even if they are solvent, they are statistically more likely to be the sole income earners in their household and/or raising a child at the same time as suffering from stress and depression. When do they get the time to properly look after themselves and detoxify? And not just of produce, but of the daily images we are bombarded with of pubescent women with clear, light, bright complexions and taut youthful skin lacking stretch marks, lumps or razor bumps.

This may lead them to reach for the quick fix approach by hiding behind foundation and eventually reaching for bleaching creams and skin lightening procedures to cover the stripping effects of some make-up. The problem is, it often has the opposite effect and exposes unsightly chokers encrusted with black spots under the neck and on the chin from plucking unattractive hair growth.

When I was a teenager, I was shocked on a blind date when on meeting my suitor at the local train station, he greeted me by stating 'I thought you were lighter'. Further into the date he also insinuated about his own use of bleaching products and enquired if I had considered doing the same. Needless to say we never dated again, but in his defence, like many young black boys, he may well have been influenced by the images of the 'exotic' light skinned women so prevalent on the MTV generation music videos.

It also wasn't the last time somebody referred to my complexion as not being quite light enough or dark enough. However, I am fortunate enough not to feel inhibited by my complexion. Furthermore, because of the powerful nature of a global media, which regularly informs us what is in and that black is often 'out', many women of colour are left with hang-ups.

Beauty is only skin deep, but as we have to wear our skin everyday of our lives, we should treasure it like our favourite black dress – dry cleaned, protected and well hung. Moreover, we need to stop trying to be superwomen, whilst itemizing looking after ourselves at the bottom of the daily 'to do' list. The illusion we create by over using cosmetics can be to the detriment of our own skin, often because we are scared to slow down in case we lose those daily battles. I have dropped my warrior mask and I feel like I have won the war.

THE DISTORTED EYE

Sheree Mack

I was in the final year of my GCSE's at Walbottle High School, an all white school in West Newcastle, when for my final English assignment I had to choose two books from the school library and write about them. It was through this task that I found *The Bluest Eye* (1972) by Toni Morrison. This was the first book that spoke to me directly, as a young black female growing up in a racist society, and what that meant to my identity and my sense of self. This was the first book that I read whose main protagonist was a black girl. Before this, I was reading *Sweet Valley High* and *Sweet Dreams* romantic novels, within which the heroine was white, blond or brunette, with blue or green eyes.

While reading, I would lose myself in the world created within the texts, high school or college, and I would always imagine myself in the position of the heroine; as white and beautiful. This is not to say that I was not proud of my blackness. I defended it against the insults to the point of drawing blood from the person who was stupid enough to call me names. This was the public face. In private, I longed to fit in and be accepted. I longed to be white. This was my double consciousness, my split personality, of being one thing and wanting to be something else. And in my imagination, I could be. I could speak with that other voice and be part of the majority of society for a change. But after reading *The Bluest Eye,* my consciousness shifted; my eyes were opened.

I remember one time I had cut my finger and my mum told me to take the plaster off to let it breathe overnight. I took the plaster off and my finger was white. I jumped for joy and shouted, 'At last I'm white'. My mum, the gentle protective one of the family, got really angry and told me never to think or say that again: I should be proud to be black. I thought then that I had done something wrong but this was forgotten in my childhood days. Until I read *The Bluest Eye,* I didn't realise I had a problem. I realised that I had been fooling myself. The predominant literature of my childhood had duped me into the belief that it was right to identify with the female lead in the book; that it was right as a young black girl that I should want to be white, popular and loved. These books allowed me to escape my reality at the same time as reinforcing the fact that I could never be white, that I could never be beautiful. However, the desire to be white was warranted through default due to the invisibility of black characters.

The Bluest Eye is about a young girl who longs to be white as then she will be seen and loved. Unconsciously, Pecola Breedlove wishes for blue eyes, '... here was a little girl asking for beauty'. She lives with her poor black family who have all suffered at the hands of white society. Her father is humiliated so many times by white men; her mother escapes her existence of looking after white families through watching films. They are a family who have no love for the self, never mind each other. This book is an example of the harsh reality of being black in a predominately white society. This book spoke to me. I was nearly sixteen years old; sixteen years too late in terms of wishing myself white, or wishing I was the same as the people I read about in the

HAIR POWER – SKIN REVOLUTION

books, that is, white and loved. It didn't matter at the time that this story was written from an Afro-American perspective. I was so green, barren and starved that this book would do; would work some kind of magic to heal the wounds.

From *The Bluest Eye,* I advanced onto other Morrison novels, *Sula, Tar Baby.* I then went onto Alice Walker, Gloria Naylor and Maya Angelou. I never thought that there were similar texts like this coming out of the British context. It wasn't until I moved to London to complete my degree in English and Geography that my personal tutor introduced me to Joan Riley and Grace Nichols. Before this, these black women writing in Britain were invisible to me.

I thought that something had to be done about this neglect and created a Black British Women's Writers' group while at Brunel University, where we, as black British women, shared what we read and educated each other about what stories, poetry and plays were out there, written by us that spoke to us. We became a supportive and encouraging network of black women readers and writers. Jackie Kay and Jean 'Binta' Breeze to name a few were invited into our university and were loved by the majority, illustrating how black women writers gain an audience through their performances, by being visible.

WRAPPED UP IN CONFLICT

Nicole Moore

Before I arrived on the scene in October 1953, tension and conflict was sitting pretty and I know this because my mother told me how her brothers in particular told her how she was quite mad and did she realise she would have black children if she married my father! Oh Mum, you knew all this and yet still in the name of love went forth into the wilderness.

So like I said, there was a nasty storm brewing even before my conception and birth. Blind intervention I call it and thank goodness I had no clue, until later on.

There was a point when I felt like an odd sock; I am not sure exactly when it was obvious except one of my uncles, Ken Hunt, used to irritate me on his visits by partly ignoring me when I opened the front door to let him in and by calling me 'Nick'. I never recall him engaging in conversation, or even small talk during my childhood – nothing except a kind of a grunt, which I guess was his way of saying hello.

Then, I internalised the uncomfortable feelings and felt voiceless to challenge my uncle's way of not greeting me and of reducing my name to what I felt was a nothing and sounded to me like a man's name. Eventually, I ignored him and I guess there was no love lost between us whatsoever. This distance with family members was something I learned to live with throughout my life. It was my way of dealing with rejection.

Of course, one could say that this was down to the times – it being the fifties – and that 'children should be seen and not heard' may have been the traditional stance at play. But, I'm pretty sure I was always entangled in a web of complex and ambiguous racial situations.

You see, I was the black sheep of the family and with an absent father, I suppose I was perceived as the result of a mad mistake my mum made. The skin I was living in, which was quite dark in my early childhood, caused quite a stir and my mum suffered not just racial abuse from within her family but when the public saw first my brown skin and then her white skin, she was called all the nastiest names under the sun, from 'nigger lover' to 'slut'. Again, I knew this because my mum told me.

Now what you have to understand is that I was oblivious to all of this although I was aware of being uncomfortable from time to time. And even though my skin tone was somehow the focus of those complex and ambiguous situations, I did not realise this at first – although I remember my grandmother referring to the African-Caribbean family who lived opposite us in our street in Highbury, North London, as 'darkies' – I did feel uncomfortable but did not have the voice or the words to respond. I kept quiet and mostly these issues washed over me.

My other Uncle Tom Hunt did engage in conversation with me and was very talented. By day, he worked in a factory and yet he was a brilliant artist. His painting of the Mona Lisa was outstanding. I always made sure to show my appreciation of this artistic streak in my uncle, much to the annoyance of his wife who was extremely jealous. She was also the most overtly racist member of our family. Here is where the beast of racism and prejudice reared its ugly head. I remember a few occasions in my childhood, when she made hurtful racist comments and so I stopped visiting my Uncle Tom when I was about 12 years old because of his wife's horrible attitude. Again, no voice; no words were expressed from my mouth and my mum never questioned why I stopped my visits. I think there was no love lost between my mum and her sister-in-law. Maybe my mum knew the real deal since the racism wasn't only expressed towards me, but indirectly to the wider society where she lived. My mum told me that my aunt, who spent most of her years living in a council flat in Stoke Newington, Hackney, London, resented those 'blacks' taking 'our' housing.

The challenges of living in my skin in an all-white household were made even more significant because I had no siblings to identify with. Growing up without any black cultural and parental influence wasn't easy and could only be substituted by a genuine desire to ensure and enjoy a balanced cultural mix of school friends. Sure, I wasn't the only child to grow up this way and now there are increasing numbers of mixed-race children in disproportionate numbers who are living in care homes and some have been adopted by white families.

To make matters worse between the ages of 13 to 20 years of age I became a foreigner from some distant land when we moved to Wellingborough, Northamptonshire, an area that was, and still is, predominantly white. Remember, this was the sixties too and those crucial teenage years were mind-blowing, especially when I left school (I couldn't wait) and tried to find work. Prejudice being the operative word meant on many occasions when I was invited for an interview after a telephone call, on arrival at reception I was told to wait, and then told 'Sorry, the job has (somehow) gone!' My skin colour was too much for those employers and when they did offer me positions they struggled worrying what the other staff members might think.

Every time I recall these events/scenarios in my mind and imagination, it raises different passions. Although there is knowledge and understanding now, these experiences mostly happened when I was less in the know and so the experience left me confused and irritated and sometimes just down right angry. It was anger at the injustice of it all and at the ignorance of a person who may have come from any walk of life whether a child, teacher, head teacher, family member and sometimes a friend, who could look at me and hold onto racist thoughts, based on my brown skin that I was living in – nothing more, nothing less.

I felt my identity was always under scrutiny and now I realise some human beings are just not good with difference; of race, culture and creed. But putting that aside, my brown skin was a real barrier or threat to white folk, as I looked different from them, so I must be different from them and on the latter, they are right. I was born a brown skinned mixed-heritage child and within that I am of course tangled up with all of those English and Guyanese ancestries and this is what the wider society perceives as different.

And all of this at a time when I was coming to terms with a loss of my multi-cultural London city friends, living in a small town in the Midlands, with its white inhabitants that didn't have a clue then what 'multi-cultural' meant and at a time when I was coming of age and starting to become interested in boys. There was a lot going on.

As I reflect here, I relive the distant experiences and wonder how I coped on a daily basis and without the maturity of life experiences. I just had to get on with the rest of my life and at times it did feel like I was living on a different planet. I had to think of innovative ways of surviving, which led to me trying on identities with strangers knowing I would never see them again.

Playing a few identity games gave me some distance and satisfaction. People to me then, seemed to want to believe I was from some distant land and when I obliged they smiled in the most satisfyingly smug way as if they knew they were right and my brown skin had a context that wasn't English/British.

From where I was standing, I knew the truth and occasionally, I would stand firm in that truth, depending on who was asking. Many times when complete strangers nosily asked me where I was from, I would make it quite clear that I was a London-born girl without the qualification of a Guyanese father and English mother. I was not always going to make what were invasions on my privacy, easy for these intruders to deal with.

Of course, these strangers sometimes left it there and looked somewhat perplexed, searching my brown skin, for a lead – an answer – and other times they reacted in a really offensive way, as if they thought I might be lying, hence the second degree questioning of 'No, where are you really from?'

Of course, human beings are curious so I totally understand how a genuinely interested person may enquire about me. But I know when that takes place because the person will ask about my cultural heritage and I will gladly oblige and tell them I was born in London and my cultural heritage is mixed – English and Guyanese.

ARE YOU BLACK OR WHITE?

Nicole Moore

Over the years, I've engaged in countless conversations and discussions relating to my mixed-heritage identity, which have mostly focused on my light brown complexion. Some of those dialogues have been meaningful with insightful musings from well-intentioned individuals who are curious about how I feel about myself and my skin, and who share their perspectives in an honest and open way.

Skin colour, in particular the hierarchy of skin shade, is a complex issue and people both black and white have a range of perspectives, depending on a variety of factors such as their race, culture, gender, class and social structure and their knowledge and experience learned – or not – along the way.

Caucasian people, mostly women, including my mother, have perceived me as 'not really black.' My Guyanese father being absent in those earlier years didn't help. Statements like, 'You're not like other black people,' or 'I don't think of you as black,' were made well before the terms racism and diversity had yet to settle into British culture. And yet, questions like 'Where are you really from?' descended upon me in strange ways when I lived in Northamptonshire, between the ages of 13 and 20. This aim to deconstruct my identity since my brown skin did not apparently qualify as 'black' and yet in the same breath I was not accepted as being born in and from London was challenging.

Caucasian people felt they had some kind of authority on the subject and all based on my skin tone and what it represented and meant to them. It was as if I existed only as whites saw me. I think this obsession with my skin tone came from fear and ignorance mainly of my claim to blackness. I slowly realised that to be black meant precisely that one was never looked at but simply at the mercy of the reflexes the colour of one's skin caused in other people. Ironically, I remember aged 17, being confronted by a mixed-race girl when I brought a Caucasian girl-friend to a West Indian dance, 'You need to make up your mind whether you are black or white', she shrieked.

As I grew stronger in my blackness, I became better equipped to take on those often challenging and sometimes irritating statements and questions. I started answering these questions with a question, making the questioner think and rethink. People started to trip over their words and I danced in delight. I developed special skills and strategies. I became more myself, who I wanted to be. The interrogators became less of an issue, more of a pest to get rid of. How dare anyone black or white or somewhere in between, assume to inform a person of colour who they are or who they are not. It's something intrusive and invasive – I have never done it myself either. Oh, I might wonder at where certain people are from but only from a point of curiousness – and I have found that curiosity, like all other desires, produces pain as well as pleasure.

As I reached my late twenties, these questions and statements almost disappeared until one day I was questioned by a three-year old Caucasian girl who attended my son's nursery in north London during the eighties. Totally out of the blue she said 'Are you black or white?' I threw the question back at her and replied, 'What do you think?' She looked at me searching for an answer, and then stared intently at my son and her smart conclusion was 'I think you are black, because you have a black son.' I became curious, so I then said, 'Well, I could be white and still have a black son.' She looked baffled and then ran off to play.

Black people, both men and women, of African-Caribbean descent, have mostly perceived me as black, although some have been naturally curious about my mixed-heritage. In fact, this kind of curiousness was standard when I met a potential black boyfriend. We would ask each other where our parents were from. Some boyfriends would also admit their preference for a light-skinned girlfriend, particularly my son's father, who was born in the UK, from Jamaican parentage. They say opposites attract, which may account for the fact that my boyfriends have tended to be dark-skinned. At the time, this didn't occur to me, but I did think my light skin and my boyfriends' dark skins complemented each other.

In June 2008 during a short trip to Jamaica, I discovered just how complex the issue of skin colour is in Jamaica, when I engaged in a meaningful conversation with a Jamaican woman called Lorraine. I was impressed with Lorraine's philosophy of life and she listened intently to my perspective and to my story; of my many trips to Jamaica and to my social interactions with Jamaican people in the UK. The most revealing element of our discussion was that in Lorraine's view, rural Jamaican people, her included, perceived my light brown skin as 'white'. Apparently, there is no real understanding of being of mixed-heritage and even when there may be some awareness, the term 'white' is still used. I wondered is that ignorance or more about how dominant 'white' is when it comes to the mixed-heritage identity?

However, Lorraine's perspective does not sum it up for

all Jamaicans. During a previous trip to Jamaica in 2007, I developed a deep and dark brown skin complexion. I was pleasantly surprised when on a few occasions, I was asked by Jamaican men, 'Which part of Jamaica are you from? 'Are you from Kingston?' This made me smile.

In December 2007, I visited Kingston for the third time and despite a short two-day visit, it was the most inspiring experience in Jamaica so far. I had been in the island for three months; long enough for me to make those cultural connections. A visit to Kingston's Rastafarian Headquarters gave me the opportunity of reasoning with sophisticated Rastafarian men and women, who welcomed and embraced me in ways that I never dreamed possible and who impressed me with their high levels of self-awareness, self-knowledge and self-understanding. I found these experiences spiritually uplifting.

Having travelled extensively all over the island of Jamaica, my favourite spot is Treasure Beach, which I have found to be the most authentically delightful and relaxing and a place where a lot of mixed heritage Jamaicans reside. Here, I blended right in, with the many fair haired, green eyed and light complexioned Jamaicans. But there is much more to this blending in. I also blended in to Jamaica's beautiful landscapes, dazzling majestic Caribbean Sea and breathtaking sunsets. I breathed in the openness of wide spaces. I was a city girl let loose in the spaciousness of it all. I learned what the term 'relaxation' really meant. As I sat feeling the ocean breeze on a daily basis, I became addicted, and wherever I looked, I saw and felt nature's power and might. Walking along the beach at sunset, I truly looked up and watched God perform those miracles that we now take for granted. As day becomes night without fail, the stars above delight us in their dance. Life to me is full of mystery and wonder.

My experience as a woman of mixed-heritage has been diverse and unique. Being born with a British nationality has no doubt dominated and dictated the perplexity of the skin I am living in. I have experienced racism in many different guises; my lighter skin didn't make any difference on those occasions. I understand that light skin is perceived as somewhat nearer to white and that light skin implies greater worth as blackness disappears drop by drop, but believe me it makes no difference, especially when you live in the UK. Having said all of this, I love my skin colour and would not want to be anything but brown-skinned.

In November 2008, Barack Obama became the first black president and yet news commentators in the UK were making statements such as 'Obama isn't black; he's as white as he is black'. For the record, Barack Obama is African-American. Let's transcend skin colour, which only keeps us in the dark. Let's stop playing with the words black and white; half black/half white. Let's talk about heritage and ancestry.

What is even more disturbing is the increasing amounts of adverts for skin lightening creams I've seen in black beauty magazines recently, which state: 'Do you want Beautiful Skin? We can lighten & brighten you to your desired skin tone without the use of harsh chemicals.' It then goes on to say, 'Rapid removal of hyper/uneven pigmentation.' Another advert states: 'Lightenex Plus – For Darker Skin Tones – The MOST Powerful Skin Lightening Cream Available!' So the ugly rejection of darkness is getting worse. European definitions of attractiveness are sweeping the non-western world too, making most populations feel envious and sometimes desperate.

So I leave you with my hopes and dreams that one day people of colour will stop whiting up and look at themselves in the mirror and love themselves first and foremost for who they are and not concern themselves with the hierarchy of skin shades. What is more important is acceptance of ourselves without measuring our beauty against Eurocentric standards.

COLOURFUL PERCEPTIONS

Cristina Odigie-Bulnes

My skin is beige in the winter and caramel in the summer. My father is a black Nigerian and my mother is a white Spaniard. If I'm asked for a label, I'll say mixed-race or biracial. I have a mixed cultural background: Spanish, English, and Nigerian. To me, my skin colour mattered enormously while I was growing up, particularly because it mattered to others.

I have a caring bond with my colour. Still, I didn't always like the skin I'm in. As a young girl, I used to fall in and out of love with it because of the unwanted attention to my looks and ambivalent questions. How my skin affects and exposes me has changed significantly along the 33 years of my life. I've changed, and so has society.

Today, I feel lucky that my skin is different. It gives me great freedom as an individual. As a kid, though, I had fleeting fantasies where my hair was straight and my skin a shade or two lighter. I hated being stared at. My fantasies of being fairer never turned into any serious wish; my family never gave me the impression that my colour was wrong.

Bleaching creams and lightening procedures are not for me. I wish people didn't find them necessary as a result of unbalanced canons of beauty around fair skin. Still, I refuse to judge those who use them as I've never been in their shoes. I don't underestimate the lasting damaging effects of colonialism, slavery, and segregation (to name a few hardships on colour.)

Times are changing. But the establishment of more contemporary aesthetic ideals will take time, consistent respect and love, and above all, a commitment to change from the media and the public.

As a kid and an adolescent, I experienced racism. But due to the lightness of my skin and my class, it was a slightly different kind of racism. Joining a clique at school break-times presented a risk. Would they be telling racist jokes again?

'Hold on a minute. My father's black. I find that joke insulting,' I'd say.

'But Cristina, you're not really black, are you?'

'Well, I'm mixed-race. I don't appreciate your sense of humour.'

It hurt terribly to be under such unfounded attacks. My family rarely acknowledged any racism because doing so would taint their view of the world. Also, due to their good standing in town, they thought I was part of the majority despite being a minority.

Growing up in an all-white town and surrounded by white family members, I too felt I belonged. Somehow I did. But I was aware that my circumstances were atypical. Talking race with my father was futile. 'Racism was an excuse to fail', he'd say. So I invested in education and academic achievement, and adhered to this colour blindness, choosing to believe that race didn't affect me. I've heard other mixed-race people say that they just live in their skin, often forgetting how they look. That's what I did.

But you can't escape a world that doesn't exactly mirror your colour. In the early eighties, there were hardly any interracial families in Vitoria, the Spanish town where we lived. My family was on friendly terms with some of them, yet a strong bond was never formed due to differences in the children's ages and interests and the families' lifestyle.

Depending on my exact location, my skin takes on a whole different meaning. In Brazil or London, for example, I blend in. In Nigeria or Spain, I don't. My colour exposes me even when I'm unobtrusive; this often required some personality adjustment to socially fit in. In my case, I was naturally shy. As I became used to being seen and being questioned about my origins, I became more social and outgoing – traits I use to my advantage now.

Moreover, my colour prompted (and still does but to a lesser degree) people to comment on my Eurocentric and Afrocentric looks and my attractiveness or lack thereof. At school, I had several male friends but was rarely asked out because of my colour. This caused wounds to my self-esteem that I later had to heal. Funnily enough, my story was that of the ugly duckling, so the tables eventually did turn.

Another by-product of my colour was that reading people became second nature. We attribute meaning and qualities to situations and people in an attempt to predict behaviour and create a sense of certainty. This human tendency of attribution is a close cousin to our need to form groups to differentiate from 'the others.' In-group and out-group dynamics – unconscious or not – are the reasons why my colour and mixedness present a puzzle to others. Hence, I've habitually met people with inept social skills and self-righteousness about my racial identity and authenticity. By just seeing my colour, individuals from all racial backgrounds assume they know my values, family history, language, class, knowledge, etc. During these social interactions, my colour gave me instant access to others' cognitive processes and assumptions about me and race.

'So what are you then?'

'Sorry, I couldn't tell you had *black* in you.'

'Please marry Black so things are fixed.'

'I'm not racist; do you think you'd be my friend if I was?'

'Why would you date a white man?'

'You must have a good scholarship to study here.'

'You went on vacation, how was the Caribbean weather?'

'Where did you learn such good Spanish?'

As a young girl, you're too vulnerable in the face of this kind of questioning. It faces you prematurely with life's crude reality. Only those in the minority truly know this experience. In Nigeria, I'm a minority too. Many members of my family resident there are accepting and loving. Yet my colour still sets off strong reactions and hurtful indirect comments, mostly among the older generations. A frightening experience with the Nigerian police, all down to my colour, temporarily put me a bit in touch with what black people have suffered, for example, in South Africa or the United States. My colour never resulted in such experiences in Spain though.

So I've met with completely different assumptions of what my colour represents. When I speak and present myself to those who've quickly labelled me, I see their assumptions crumbling at the same speed as my self-expression. The changes in their body language and facial gestures rarely conceal their surprise. I've seen this happen particularly once they meet me after having established a long-term professional relationship over the phone and email. Generally, I've had little problems and, on the whole, relationships have carried on fine.

However, I know my colour affects me as a minority. This is why I befriend respectful, multicultural and racially intelligent individuals who reflect my inner reality. Professionally and personally, my colour and experiences induce me to observe and monitor people's racial comfort zones.

I didn't always live in Spain. I was born and raised in England for over six years. My mother tells me she realised that both my brother's and my colour would unfairly work against us in seventies and eighties England. She'd noticed passing remarks from teachers and blatant racism portrayed in the media. In 1982, wanting to protect us from the self-fulfilling destiny that England had in store for us, my parents decided that the family should relocate to Vitoria, Spain, where my mother's middle-class family lived.

Spaniards are known for their darkness, which is a result of their Moorish past. One would think the remains of such an historic ethnic influence would diminish the extent of racism there, but that was (and still is) not the case. My father was generally liked by my mother's large family, but I have little doubt that I would have been loved considerably less if I had been born with a darker complexion. But my father's a doctor. If my father's class and my colour had been different, maybe I would be writing a whole different story today.

We mixed-race individuals tend to look different at various stages of life, and you'd be surprised to see how dissimilar I've looked along the years. A simple sojourn at the beach, a new hairstyle, or a mere change of hair colour can blur the racial boundaries of people's perceptions of my ethnicity. When I began straightening my hair in my mid-twenties, I passed for white too often. Since I've returned to my curls, there have been fewer doubts about my mixedness.

By my own initiative I've travelled to Nigeria, and I try to keep in contact with some of my family there. Still, I'd wished my family – mostly my Nigerian father – would have tried harder to expose me to the other half of my ethnicity.

Today, I integrate and celebrate my colour and

uniqueness. The learning and multicultural experiences provided by my colour are irreplaceable and invaluable. For example, I'm a skilled social shifter, with dual loyalties and multiple cultures. My rich inner life is regularly stimulated and challenged by others. The ability to see both sides of the story means I'm a natural mediator. Also, I choose to feel whiter or blacker depending on my feelings and reactions to a situation. I'm good at observing people's beliefs and intentions through their language, questioning, and reactions.

Granted, I make swift faulty judgements based on looks just like everybody else, but as a result of the bittersweet experiences around my colour, I have a good enough social and racial intelligence, which enables me to think twice before I talk.

Well, most of the times.

BEYOND THE SKIN WHERE NO MIRROR CAN REFLECT

Akuba Quansah

I remember when I was invited by the Southall Caribbean Parents Group (West London) in the late seventies, at the tender age of seventeen years old to contribute to a conference on the theme of **'Black Youth in British Society'**, against the backdrop of the Southall race riots in the aftermath of the killing of New Zealand teacher, Blair Peach. After reciting some poems I had written specially for the event I gave a presentation on what it felt like for me being 'black' in Britain, which unavoidably led me to unveil first to the audience my own early childhood experiences, in particular those primary, first five years of my life that would shape how I perceived who I was and the different relations and relationships I would have in years to come. I spoke of being an only child, of Ghanaian parentage, that I was born in West London in 1962 and that my mother – who was then studying to be a nurse and my father, who travelled around the world with the shipping liner, the Black Star Line, as a radio/radar officer- had jointly decided to have me privately fostered out to a white family in Essex, as I later realised, of English working class heritage, where I stayed from around three months old to about six years old. This was to offer my parents a temporary solution to the childcare problems they faced as professional working parents who were new migrants to Britain with no extended family support systems to assist with my care.

Within this biographical context I nervously explained to a rather impassioned-looking audience, with one or two exceptions, how, as a young six year old, and even younger, I did not understand what 'being black' meant in any real cultural or political sense because in this foster family set up there were no conversations about my African background and culture, no talk about my blackness or more appropriately about 'colouredness' since anyone of African origin in the idiom of 1960s racial talk in Britain could only be described as 'coloured'. Unsurprisingly, there was also a collusion of silence about who my natural parents were, I expect, because any discussion with me about my family genealogy would have unavoidably impelled my foster carers to confront and deal with the factor of me being 'coloured'.

One male member of the audience, in a rather derisory and inquisitional tone, responded, "What do you mean you did not know you were black, could you not see that your skin looked different to everyone around you when you looked in the mirror?" His question provoked raucous laughter, at my expense, which cut real deep, and I stood silently quivering, frozen and somewhat intimidated as I had somehow assumed a gladiatorial role, not knowing how to respond to what seemed, for a few excruciatingly painful seconds, to be a very poignant point. A few seconds was all I needed to regain my perspective and the confidence to put that particular questioner diplomatically yet firmly in his place.

"How could I know from looking in the mirror that my skin was black and that my identity was black African when I was conditioned to be colour – blind?" The tables had now turned, and as I lapped up the head–nodding and claps of acknowledgment from most of the audience, it was now this male inquisitor who felt under siege. The truth is, though I did not show it, I knew inwardly that several emotional chords had been struck that would take a short period of stay in Ghana and years of personal introspection and social-anthropological study to help me make full sense of. The fact is that at 17 years old 'being a young black female' living in London represented for me sheer cultural confusion and conflict, which was played out deeply within the epidermis of my skin, a conflict that had plagued me from my primary years right through to my thirties.

At age six years old in 1966, my parents decided the time was right to reclaim me from the domicile clutches of my foster carers for the purpose of taking me to Ghana, on board one of the Black Star Line ships my father navigated, to discover and learn about my African heritage, roots, culture, language, 'blackness', yes the whole works. Strangely enough, I have no memory of my initial reaction to encountering my *real* mother and father at the foster parents' home as they arranged for my leaving but I do remember being on a ship that was about to disembark from London Docks, with two families. One of these families claimed to be my 'mummy and daddy' whom I did not know but whose skin colour began to fascinate and puzzle me and the other, whom I had known for the first six years of my life as 'Nanny and Father Clowe', whose skin colour suddenly became noticeable to me along with that pained look of sadness, probably, as I have come to reflect later, over having to give me up. That having to give me up was simultaneously the beginning of a long process of exfoliating layers of an assumed white identity through being raised by a white English family who were incapable of 'talking black'. Unwittingly or wittingly my newly acquired biologically related parents had planted the seeds of curiosity in me that propelled me to notice racial and culture difference, albeit rather simplistically, for the first time by virtue of the fact that they had a different colour of skin to my foster parents, which was akin to my own colour of skin, and spoke a different language ('Nzema') unfamiliar to me as well as ate a variety of food different to what I had been used to (yam, plantain, 'fufu' with light, pepper soup, jellof rice and so on), and even wore a type of clothing (especially my mother) that looked different to what I was used to seeing on the Clowe family or local people in Essex.

On the ship journey to Ghana at night in the cabin I shared with my mother, when she undressed in my presence, I vividly remember being so magnetised by the appearance of her 'dark' and smooth – feeling skin that I would often smell and feel parts of her body like her arms and legs as I laid beside her. From the first day of being in my mother's parental care she introduced me to the daily ritual of creaming her body, from head to toe, with a sweet scenting oil or pomade after showering as a necessary African practice to help keep our skin smooth and shiny in texture. Unused to this process of 'creaming the skin' and it's seemingly rejuvenating effects, I really enjoyed feeling and smelling her body. In contrast her hair did not fascinate me quite as much because she tended to cover the tightly bounded threaded hairstyle she wore with a scarf at night or with an Europeanised-looking wig during the day.

When our ship finally arrived at Takoradi Docks in Ghana, and as I stepped out of the enormous vessel with my parents, first feeling the sweltering heat like nothing I had ever experienced before, I could not help but stare at the hoards of people who passed by. They were speaking in dialects I did not understand, and women and children, mostly, wearing a variety of colourful, patterned style of clothing I had only seen before worn by my mother on the ship. People passing by stared at me too and, as I clung tighter to my mother's hand whilst my father arranged for some transport to take us to our destination, I wondered why I was being stared at. After all, I thought to myself, 'isn't my skin colour brown like the people passing me by in the streets? When I asked my father why people continued to look at me he explained that even though I had come back to my country of origin, local Ghanaians regarded me as a 'white' English person because I was born and raised in England, spoke only English with an English accent, and most illuminating of all, because my skin was lacking a certain tone and tan that comes with living in a hot, tropical country like Ghana and which local inhabitants can easily distinguish.

In Ghana, I assumed I no longer suffered from colour-blindness; I now saw my skin as brown, yet to other Ghanaians, whether at school, or in the vicinity, they regarded me as a 'white' Ghanaian girl. It would take years to find that equilibrium of seeing myself as a 'British born black woman of Ghanaian descent.' Looking in a mirror could never have been enough for me to have acquired a concrete sense of my cultural identity. I have had to look into my inner self, deep beyond the skin, to find the true me within.

POEMS: HAIR

Settling In

Mid-thirties, and I settle into myself
like sitting in an armchair that has sat
in the corner, faded and scruffy,
unnoticed for too long;
decide I'm not so bad after all, with
my big thighs and well-worn
still-soft mocha-brown skin
fat knees passed down the generations,
tooth from my mother
that has stuck out in photos
over the years like a fang,
the hair that has been compared
to sheep's wool, and the rest;
my face, that in spite of it all
still looks fresh, and young,
the arms that are not sinewy and toned
but have carried children alone
and cleaned, and cleaned!
I decide I will never be the tiny- waisted
girl with the long blonde hair
and the golden smile
and the legs like a gazelle
that go on for miles
that I always wanted to be,
and settle for seeing the beauty in me.

Louisa Adjoa-Parker

Me and my 'fro

Me and my 'fro
Nappy, natural
Dense, defending
Strong, pretending
Me and my 'fro

Me and my 'fro
Head high
Posture of pride
Balanced inside
Me and my 'fro

Me and my 'fro
Claimed back position
Everlasting transmission
A supply of inspiration, transformation and still irritation
Me and my 'fro

A gesture for communication
A love-declaration
A Self-embracing
Me and my 'fro

Gennett Aku Agbenu

No Lye!

Clasped between our mother's knees,
We sit patiently,
Afro comb, hair oil and comb.
Back and bottom aching,
As our hair is pulled
And stretched into submission.

Clasped between our mother's knees,
We sit patiently,
Waiting for corn rows, twists or plaits.
Wanting to touch,
But fearing the comb slap.
Our pride and honour in our hair.

Clasped between our mother's knees
We sit, dreaming of when
Our hair was soft, shiny and curly.
Waiting for ribbons, beads
Hair bands and clips
To adorn our crown.

Clasped between our mother's knees
We learn about good hair; bad hair;
Pretty hair; picky hair.
Mixed messages of inferiority based on
An, "I am better than you",
Value System.

But when I am grown
And released from my master's knees
My mind will be free to embrace and reclaim who I am.
And my beauty will not be defined
By the wig, the weave
Or the Lye.

Scherin Barlow Massay

Hair We Are

Shirley wanted her hair straight nice and straight like her friend
She'd tried tonging and ironing it and it STILL refused to bend.

"Shanice's hair moves when she shakes her head like this
Why's mine stay the same?"
"Ah, our hair's wild and her hairs thin and tame
Better to have neat rows of cane than use relaxer-
Damage yuh hair bad baad.
Jheri curls the thing anyway now relaxer's just a fad"

"What yuh chat bout Monique it's 1989
Michael Jackson dropped the wet look long loong time!
Jheri Curl's a curse anyway, everyone knows where yuh been
Got caught out nuff times, too many places my grease stains been seen
If that wasn't bad enough, parents can hear yuh comin'
Too much "drip drip" come like a tap been left running!"

"Yuh chattin' rubbish Shirley, it's all about the *natural* look
I'd rather be true to my hair than false like a crook
I like my kinks and patterns; they make me individual
That straight hair gal Shanice, she's just a smooth criminal
Get over Michael Jackson girl, he's hardly Mr. Natural
Yuh wanna get deep, I'll hit you with something factual
Our hair grows towards the sky, cos we are children of the sun"

"Who the hell told you that?!"
"Don't dis it comes from me mum!"
"Oh...."

"Yuh know we're kind of lucky y'know Shirley cos we can choose so many styles

One day we can bus weave the next, bus it out wild!"

"Y'know I guess your right Shirley, none of them are right or
wrong
I love the "natural look" me but some days I like to tong"

"I love being a woman, being unique creative and fresh
Being changeable chameleons, changing one day to the next"

"Your tellin' me my God, I really think it's great
Especially as I can change my hair for every date!"

Daniella Blechner

Accept me, for me

I've had the straight style
The curly perm too
Had the false extensions
For way too long

My hair journey started
From an early age
With the hot comb press
And the tingeing of ears

Then came the curlers
Could not sleep at night
They were bulky and hard
No sleep for the wicked

The curly perm had
My scalp and pocket in spasms
With the amount of oils
That kept my hair so shiny

There came a time
When I realised that
I am still beautiful naturally
With what God gave me

I followed my instincts
Deserted the media hype
Now the world has no option but
To accept me, for me!

Christine Collymore

My Hair

Why oh why is my hair so thick?
Honestly it takes the mick
Sometimes the comb breaks in my hair
So I have to give it a lot of love and care
It's tight and curly
Really girly
When it's wet it goes all floppy
When I run my hand through it's so sloppy
I like it when it's in a pom pom
I usually get it done by my mum
People tell me I should get it relaxed
But I prefer to use my old bee wax
Deep deep down I really love it
Because its mine and it makes me shine!!!!

Leaya Collymore

Jan Blan Hair

du Boulay my name
Yeah that's French
Not a slave name I add in my defence
Of bronze brown skin
Jan blan hair
Afro-Amerindian
Chabin air

Hybrid black
Attitude black
Synthesised black
A Diaspora black
A displaced 'impure' uncompromising black
Like Angela Davis
Even though I've got hair
Like Langston Hughes

Should I
Communicate perhaps
Interchangeably
In three languages maybe
Yoruba, Creole and English
Would illustrate perfectly
A more precisely triple identity

That could adapt
As per your whim
A triple identity
That once stacked into
Disparate sections
Would render me
Less threatening
Less confusingly exotic
Softer
More gamely
More specifically erotic

But instead
I take my not very dark body
And go cruise
Find a muse
And with chromatically dark acceptance I
Lose myself
In the colours of the blues...

Dorothy Cornibert du Boulay

Mi Face or Mi Hair

Well mi hair is a constant wonder to others
Some call it good hair and others say it look like wig
There is a constant amazement how mi nu do nuting to it and it
still stay good
Like is my fault mi mix up mix up
Mi nuh wash it unless it necessary and mi nuh trouble it if it
nawh trouble me
Mi sorry if it upset yu but never mind
If it wasn't mi hair
It would a bin mi face
So mek me tek time and gwan wid mi hair!

Karron Francis-Darling

Curly Sue

My hair is a reflection of me
Wild, crazy and free

With little curls or ringlets, that bounce and move
A modern day look , I've got the groove

Being mixed race my hair without products, will be frizzy.
Not keen on an afro, or shaggy perm, it would drive me crazy.

Curly hair, light skin and big hooped earrings, I can be
mistaken for Latino
Not black, white or Filipino

I've been asked would you like your hair straight?
Everyone wants a different look, you'll see, just wait.

I'm happy with the curls I've got
Maybe dressing more ethnic, might give it a shot.

I'd like to try little canerows,
Having extensions, when I get the dough
I love the idea of highlights and lowlights
Never blonde or blue black, with those colours I'd look a sight.
My skin tone doesn't suit strong colours.
Choosing foundation, can take hours.
The texture of my hair is dull and dry
No matter how much conditioner or gloss, not sure why

Hairstyles are limited and few
Controlling my curls is hard to do
But I wouldn't swap them that's for sure
Just need to experiment a few times more

Legandra Gebrakedan

Hair Place

This unrelenting task with hand brush clasped
Drawn far from grace from cuts of curls
Of streaming lace in tip top snatches
The comb strikes fierce by each brush stroked
It won't go through, swept again
I pull and tack, heave it through the back
Stuck fast in this head hitting lock of knots

Ow, ow, ow, Eeeeeazy

No stopping this knotting, tired arms flopping
The body's top lot keeps me tugging at clumping
Unstable hair pretending to exist in an always
Tiresome disentangle, wanting to get trimming
My hair down to nothing, desiring the same pressure
That GI Jane has cooking but I keep brushing
And brushing until I am entirely unknotted.

Nicola Greenwood

Happy ending

the longest
thickest braid
known connects
every black
woman's tender
scalp to
a universal pair
of burnt honey
hands that belong
to your mama.

folklore does a perfect
front flip, then eases
down into a sunny
something that doesn't
ever hurt.

she works
from the root
and understands
bergamot, her knuckles
tingle with the heat
of heavy historical
references on why
you are beautiful.
footnotes in her fingers
greasing grace all
through the tough parts.

Zakia Henderson-Brown

Long story

relax it
as if
it were
   upset.

cotton
stamped
mean
on the
scalp
like a
warning,
a war,
grown from
the inside
out.

as if
some state
of emotional
turmoil
caused it
   to coil.

consider
it a natural
defense;
a site
of organic
protest;
god's small
proud strategy,
anything
but retreat.

calm
it down
      your back.

burn
the roots
into peace,
the wild ends
     into place.

the little
compass in
your purse,
spinning

then still,
then: do
not over
think this,
then: just
stop.

Zakia Henderson-Brown

Great Hair or Great Sex? You Can't Have Both!

Great hair or great sex, you can't have both.
Well you can but just not at the same time
and certainly not if you have hair like mine.
Mine is a mane that's hard to tame.
It's a chore that I'll forever endure.
It's a long process and so much more.
More like a journey or even a mystery tour.
You see my hair has a life of its own,
which morphs even if you leave it alone.
At times I just let nature take its course,
as it's all natural of course.
If you prefer, call it virgin hair as it is otherwise known.

Growing up as a child,
I didn't give my hair much thought.
I was more interested in swimming
and all sorts of sports.
I was a right little tomboy,
blissfully playing without a care.
My mum had the task of doing my hair
which at times was a bit of a nightmare.
Only now can I fully understand her despair.
It's a great feat to maintain my mane.
Every month it takes up to twenty one hours,
which some would call insane.

Please believe me that I'm really not vain.
Although at times I feel my efforts are in vain,
when it starts to frizz up in the rain.
(I guess I should be more like Rihanna, anna, anna, eh, eh).
My hair is dark brown, long and very, very thick,
which is where the problem kicks in.
Most styles are hard to sustain, straight hair is hard to contain,
within an hour it would expand to a Tina Turner type do

and eventually morph into a great big afro if left to its own devices. Having it tied up in a bun, really isn't much fun, and the afro is quite retro. I'll leave that to the too cool for old skool hip hop bro's. Having my hair in twists is the only way to go, more to the point it's the only way I know, so if you have any other suggestions let me know, I look forward to hearing what your advice is.

Tracy Henry

Scarlet
(First published in *RED*, 2010)

As you sculpt your supple locks into an ample crest
I keep one eye on you and the other on the hope that you'll join
me
Take rest from your tireless task to let each dappled vine spill
from the chalice of your mane like tamarind husks
Descending.
Descending among you
Descending among me
Until I shall wear them like garlands,
Sun blushed and coiled neatly around the ashen canvas of
bare foot and wrist in a poultice of relic twine
A crush of crimson flex that quickens my slackened pulse
within two beats of my instinct to think.......
.......to sink deeper into the thickets bare, till I am nothing but
a shoal of silver fish now, piercing through cutlets of lobe and
brow as I too
Become estranged into your swarm.

Louise Hercules

Divine Dreadlocks

Africa is wrapped around my dreadlocks.
I'd love to swap my trainers and socks
for sandals and sunshine...
We all need to 'let go' some time.
These days, there's no hairdressing bill to pay
and the mornings of brushing and combing have melted away.

I hear the sweet voice of dreadlocks calling.
Opening the curtains to freedom each morning
is a reality that pleases me, and I belong.
In this strange land I sing my own song.

We need to escape from western faith:
Gonna wash my heavy natty-dready in The Nile.
I did away with the chemicals; replaced it with *natural style!*
I'm mixing Aloe Vera with the sap from sugar cane.
Soothing my black-brown locks in tropical rain.
I'm natural, wild, and free once again.

Michelle Hubbard

Rollers

She took her time to tame her mass of hair.
First, she'd make a strong mug of tea and sit
at the high teak table with a plastic bag.
Her cigarette smoke would claim the air.

A long wide comb in a cup of water,
she'd pull it out, tapping off loose droplets,
before running the comb through her thin hair.
The comb would straighten out the grey black frizz.

Still holding the sections, comb back in the cup,
she'd take a pink roller out of the bag
and start at the tips of her hair, rolling
upwards and under.

Only a pink and black sausage roll
was left in her hand ready for a grip,
like a white overcoat, encased the roll.
She'd take a sip of tea and a quick drag.

Then she'd take the comb again, wet and pull
on her tangled locks until it was straight.
Rollers would be rolled up and under
and covers in place, again and again,

until her whole head was a mass of rows.
Pink and white rolls, like gums and teeth,
gradually drying, gradually curling
straight. After Sunday dinner and dishes done,

the rollers would be pulled out swiftly.
These relaxed curls were then teased out like notes
from a saxophone, until they danced around
her head like a lion's mane but tamed.

Sheree Mack

I am my hair

Like Samson, I drew my strength from my locks.
In their duality, soft kinky keys that sit atop my head.
Standing above my shoulders in their afro stance.
Proud – my hair, my beauty, won't let Delilah too close with her shears,
As she nears, my ends, I split!

Cut loose, my hair bounces – dancing in front of the mirror once blown dry.
Reincarnated, post that eighties 'wet look' the shampoo had recreated.
Recoiling when wet like a spring; but now it has sprung.

Oiled, my tresses recall days of youth when sat between mum's knees.
Scalp parted like a hot cross bun.
Hair plaited sweetly into quarters.
The *Dax* that missed the scalp hit the legs.
But that was the primary look.

Secondary Septembers saw conking not conkers, but there was no relaxing when straightened, 'nappy less', baby hairs receded
– a fate no jam or spritz could abate...
...As if some punishment for rejecting your curls and tipping hats to Madame Walker.
'Good' hair gone bad – now forced to hide under wigs.
Should have went for the jheri curl like the others or stuck to the hot comb.
Reading Sophisticates Black Hair, we all embraced the canerows, twists and braids like brandy.
Like liquor, it again became cool to plait – to be re-entangled in this extension of your culture.

Collegiate: the eight hours of braiding was averted.

It was time to bob like Monica, one of those days to find some other cultural symbol.

Busy, we slipped into the ease of steams, wraps and flat irons, the smell of singed hair the nasal signature accompanying our attempts to get that Aaliyah side sweep.

Weaving our way through life, celebrating our hair from root to tip, in rainbow colours no headscarf could hide.

Like a bald headed eagle India seeks to soar – for she is *not* her hair.

Setting trends where Solange and Cassie follow, young rappers cry that girls should not look like guys.

But like our brothers; our hair makes statements with, or without, our consent.

They may fade, hit high-tops or let doo-rags set 'S-curls', but Africa's men *and* women are locked in a thick and woolly shared hair-ritage full of mystique and intrigue.

Whether Barbershop or Beauty shop; our hair tells tales of who we are *and* who we are not.

Fiona Mckinson

My Hair

My hair has had an amazing life; I've put it and myself through real stress and strife. In the early years as a child with a small voice, it was always kept short, 'So it looked neat,' my mum said. In my early teens, I sang out and cried 'I want long hair Mum!' It grew out at the sides. I loved my afro.
As part of the seventies 'Black is Beautiful' era,
My natural hair grew wild and free and all I used
in between weekly washes was an afro comb and oil sheen on my tresses.

But I felt the need to experiment, like all young women do
You name it I tried every 'fashionable' style I knew. The curly perm took the eighties by surprise; my hair grew lengthways and soon reached my shoulders. I really thought I had arrived. Little did I realise the perilous journey my hair was embarking upon and it got worse...
In the early nineties, my eager to please hairdresser, Denise, relaxed my then natural tresses

And here was the most unnecessary of all my hair stresses, which I paid good money for on a monthly basis.
Now I have to admit a breakthrough came in the name of Eva – the beautician who told me that she could blow dry my hair instead of resorting to chemicals. This was a cool breakthrough but I still needed regular trips to the hairdresser.
And when I moved away from Eva's knowledge and expertise

I was led into the valley of destruction by a demon who relaxed
my hair taking any hint of life right out of each and every
follicle on my head. Its lifelessness just lay down completely flat
and dead. 'Never again,' I said, as I took special measures to
repair the chemical damage on my head. There was only one
thing for it a series of steam treatments followed by a shorter
chic style while patiently awaiting new growth. The months
passed by and I took what I believe was a lesser risk.

Relaxing had had its day – and a new texturising technique
had come into play, but before this journey into the unknown, I
took a gap year and became Ms Braids, Ms Extensions, still on
an experimental road, with human wavy hair of blonde, beige
and brown shades, which if I was lucky lasted two months. The
price to pay was the length of time it took – the best part of a
day and even longer taking them out. The effects were instant
long hair...and I discovered blondes did have more fun!

The journey continues and I have returned full circle
to a natural free and liberating style,
which three years on, has reached great lengths.
I love my locs and they are here to stay as they are connected
not only to my head but also to my African-Caribbean cultural
ancestry.

Nicole Moore

Hair on my head

With growing hair on my head they may stare
but with the desire of it we can only just do our 'do' how we want
to
why is it desired?
it can be hired
at a price it makes you look nice, some people think twice and
wonder is it hers?
some love to run fingers through it
massage it
wash it
everyday
until it resembles hay
or lovely locks to go with frocks
that hair of mine I say
get out of bed
and dye it red
braid it, twist it, wrap it or cut it, cornrows you say, just for today
don't want my hairline to take the strain
kinky, afro, yeah get to it, black is beautiful don't you know it!
rejected for so long with that straightening comb, flinching every
minute
from the source, authentic, not stringy
your hairs so thick "I wish I had it" they say
oh how I dismay about our crowning glory
every strand tells a story

Bola Odeyemi

HAIR POWER – SKIN REVOLUTION

It's only hair today....gone tomorrow

Three packs of false hair on my head, so now I can get out of bed
I'm a get up and go sista, facing the new world, having hid my tight curls
the day before I ditched the 'fro, I just want to get up and go
feeling accepted
no longer rejected
by people and places, jumping to conclusions
about the kinky hair I choose to move with
natural I was politicised
weaved up I'm beautified
I ask myself, why does my 'fro carry both symbolism and criticism?
connotations of militancy, weaved up I am all femininity
always asked "what are you gonna do to your hair" by sistas as they stare
as if my afro is an unfinished work in progress hairstyle
but I'd rather walk a mile on hot coal
than be told I'm relaxing that unmanageable hair
I've come so far in my emotional journey
to not have that put on me
OK mum you didn't want to deal with it, but I, my hair and my bright African print headscarves will
no one better tell me they think it ill
now I feel like a sell out with my sewn in tracks
patting not really scratching is part of the weave
take this shit out
I want my 'fro back PLEASE!

Bola Odeyemi

HAIR

(First published in *Hair: A Journey into the Afro and Asian Experience*, 2006)

Haveityourway
Anystyleyouwant
Inseasonoutofseason
Reflectionofyourself

Elayne Ogbeta

Rapunzel, Rapunzel

(First published in *Hair: A Journey into the Afro and Asian Experience*, 2006)

Rapunzel, Rapunzel, my beauty so rare
Please will you let down your fine relaxed hair?

Oh no, dear Prince, I can't, I'm afraid,
For today I'm having my hair done in braids.

Rapunzel, Rapunzel, my beautiful maid
Can you please let down some of your braids?

Oh no, dear Prince, but would you believe!
On my dark head, I'm having a weave.

Rapunzel, Rapunzel, you I'll never leave.
Please will you let down your wonderful weave?

Oh no, dear Prince, Oh please don't squirm.
'Cause today I've decided to have me a perm.

Rapunzel, Rapunzel my love I affirm
Can you please let down your ravishing perm?

Oh no, dear Prince, I could slap my wrist.
Did I not mention that I'm having a twist?

Rapunzel, Rapunzel, in my dreams I have kissed.
Please will you let down your elegant twists?

Oh no, dear Prince, I'm ever so slow.
I forgot to tell you that I'm having a 'fro.

Rapunzel, Rapunzel, am I not your beau?
Could you please let down your soft afro?

Alas! Dear prince but we cannot be wed.
The truth is my love, there's no hair on my head.

Elayne Ogbeta

Hair Speaks slavery

Strands of soft, silky, curly locks,
Kweku's hair embodied
Centuries of conversations
Along racial lines,
That unquestionably defined identity
As worthy or unworthy of respect
By those who erected this hierarchy.

"Oh Gracie, your baby has good, *coolly* hair!
Don't you dare locks it up, you hear!"
The message was loud and clear.
Slavery had certainly left its mark.
For more than four hundred years,
And few blacks of African descent
With varying textures upon our heads
Would be spared such racist evaluations.

A European comb became a useful tool,
For the enslaver to assess
How more or less black his purchase was.
A comb that combed with much ease
Was sure to please the owner,
Who usually assigned his slave?
A lighter workload.

If Kweku's silky curly locks
Was seen by some to be positively good,
By implication then my hair,
'Locksed' and freed up of chemical wares,
Could only be negatively bad,
And even though my hair seemingly fails
To uphold strands of whiteness,
I could not care less,
Because having 'Afro textured hair'
Is something I am profoundly proud to stress!

Akuba Quansah

Hairdresser: Budapest!

The "Welcome! Afro & Euro hair!"
sign of the Nigerian's salon in Budapest,
calls out – my hair answers back.
Wearing my locks, only on the inside now,
outside my naked hair is keener, sharp.
Uncombed potential, tightly curling
with the air's moisture,
with the sweat out my skin -
my hair answers back.

The tall River State woman dives in
my raw hair. With your hands
on my head, take your time
bring me to fullness, slowly.
Fingertips first, you find my roots,
the warmth of them on my scalp.
As you conduct rising heat,
all tension peels away:
I let slip, a deep sigh, let slip a deep smile.
Sweetwater running down
each strand, to pool in
each follicle, and from there to
another plane, flooding
my chakra – a fountain sparkling.
My hair is glorious in your palms,
a duet to my cloud, tenderly at prayer.
In worship, down under my ends,
you tickle tracing circles, you knead
my undergrowth and I rise up in your chair,
now a throne, for my godhead.

Hairdresser – with your hands,
you bring me out of myself.
Comb, trim, dress and shape me
to my own contours, with room to grow.
Dreadlocks inside, raw hair outside.
Keen potential, loose to the atmosphere.
My hair answers back,
every blade of my mane,
singing.

Dorothea Smartt

Hairdresser: holding her own

My hair will answer back, but never
to the heat of a comb, scorching
chemicals stripping her straight, to lie
limp and languid. Until she,
malleable, tangible barometer,
revives herself in a fine rain's spray,
or the humidity of the day.
Shape coming in waves, like ripples
the sea leaves on sand.
My roots undulate, tightening curls.
In salt, fresh, or coconut water, each twist a cup.
Suspended like a cloud. Defying gravity
my hair springs up, and out!
Holds herself. Holds her own.

Dorothea Smartt

Hairdresser: tender partings

Tiny tangled ringlets will part -
to the gentle edge of a opening comb.
I revert, back to tender mornings:

Mummy. On a Barbados morning, away
from vacation fingers sea salt taken hold of my hair,
leading to a problem-solving barbershop call!

A beach morning, friendly-brother Jewish father,
hands practicing for your daughters' critical mass,
wild, alternative, a sign of a good home.

Daddy. On school mornings. doing his best
remembering from daughters before
to tidy a fraying braid, set ribbons to rights.

In these kind hands, even my neck-
back hair is human, right, well-behaved
and damn good hair!

Dorothea Smartt

POEMS: SKIN

My Skin Tells a Story

My skin tells a story
It began with a once
And remained forever
Grazes of spots
Darkened and scarred
Travelling in herds
Across skin
In response to life's interior juices
What could they do?
As the years grew older
The spots needed a companion
And the skin did answer
With hair, black, thin, and sharp
Blades like black grass
Formed on neck, sides and chin
And the surface in between remained brown
Longingly I wished it to cover and hide
Blades of hair and darkened spots
Where is the skin I wish to honour?

Marcellina Aderibigbe

Mulatto Girl

See the mulatto girl walking
down country lanes and fields, her
head held high, her skin the colour
of caramel boiling on the stove. See her smile
in the knowledge she is not the first
to walk this green and pleasant
countryside, she has history stirring within her limbs.
she has Africa's heat and England's cold rain
pumping through her blood, her
DNA a beautiful mix of gene pools
scattered across continents, she is strong.
She shows Africa in a way the English hide.
She shows an eighteenth century master's love for slaves.
She shows a slave's contempt.
She shows twentieth century people brave enough
to cross a line made of different tones of skin,
to love in spite of hate.

See the mulatto girl walking
down country lanes and fields, her head
held high, her quadroon baby girls
held on her hips, her hair thick and frizzed, lips
half full, there are no
white men dressing her in robes and jewels,
but see her smile, see her sway, her head
held high as she walks.

Louisa Adjoa-Parker

U HEAP of skin

Unique in
>Fitting my mass and size
>Its ability to heal and regenerate
>Elasticity and forming of stretch marks
>Accompanying me through thick and thin
>Relating my stories of beauty and health

Holding in
>A multitude of unbroken bones
>Countless highways of blood vessels
>Attachments of clinging, resistant fat
>My survival kit of essential organs
>All this, every single day of my life

Exposed to
>The temperatures of the continents
>Striking rays of ultraviolet A and B
>Moistening effects of heaven's blessings
>Friction of natural and manmade textiles
>Touches of others, accidentally or lovingly

All over
>Shades of ancestral inherited colour
>The variation in silky smoothness
>Occasional markings of trophy scars
>Raised peaks of minute pimples
>With age the speckling of darkened moles

Perceptions of
>Indication of years on this earth
>Predictor of current and future wellness
>Knowledge of ancestral inheritance
>Can you really know me from the outside?
>There's soul in my heap of skin

Christine Collymore

Black

Black, you may think of
Darkness and being alone
Dirt in a small little hole
Plain does not do anything
Dark so deep within

But when I think of black I think of
Smartness, always there on special occasions
Fun, always something different
Power, to give us a fair chance
But most of all, I think of me and my personality

Leaya Collymore

Tuareg indigo

I am she who wears colour on skin
Adorning flesh with desert shades of indigo
My stories tell themselves below eyes
Above buttered cheeks
I have no need for a metal sky
A casket carved of bone, mortared in blood
I am a million constellations moulded of mud
The colour of a waking sky
Purple blue memories, sand storm covered secrets
Between my lover the desert
And I

Tjawangwa Dema

Diaspora: Souvenirs from the edge

These are the contents of her purse
It sequoia brown, faded leather
With strips of off white threading
Keeping the old bag together

She keeps with herself an old diary
Numbers and names of people
She does not know anymore
Blue inked scribbles leaning urgently
To the edges of the page
Bright red lipstick borrowed but never returned
A face smiles back, snapshots of a life forgotten
Or not remembered every day anymore
Cards with fading logos and edges
Chewed off by time and touch
Most mornings the keys find
A corner in her purse
To snuggle and snag on what little paper there is
Receipts she does not need to keep
And cards that stopped paying
The day she stopped living their way
Today keys cuddled in palm
Fingers running through long ago coloured hair
The knob turns steady in trembling hand
Then stills as life mimics art
On shiny tiled floor the snapshot half comes to life
Remembering she has only herself to blame
Only herself to her name

That these are the contents of her life
Her skin sequoia brown, tough weathered leather
Strands of greying almost white feathers for hair
Her fading memory
The only thing keeping her today and yesterdays together
Tjawangwa Dema

Interpretation

Before I emerged into the entirety of me
Before I grew into the dappled folds and
Softened flanks of the ripened swell

I was once another

A taut buttocked high thighed creature
Firmed with meagre breasts and eyes
Wired to disarm battalions with the

Whispered slight of me

With a bounty of silken curls lacquered
In the scent of autumnal fruits
Of berry, of quince of honeyed plum

All awash a ravened flock

That fed and billowed across
My face as I strengthened
The core of my stance

But now, now I have changed

And they have settled into the crisp
Oyster froth which frames me
Casts me in an unfamiliar text

That absorbs me as I become, yet another.

Louise Hercules

Skin Layer

In the room by myself
With the TV on
In the background.
I put my laptop to use,
Whilst I look at my skin
And note how smooth
It is and how I feel calm.

But soon enough,
A memory emerges
Of how different it can be,
When you are here with me
And the texture of my skin
Gradually changes
To goose pumps.

I feel tension in my head.
I guess because I dread
To think of the possibility
Of you getting under my skin,
Like an invasion when you

Simply wish to win the argument
By personal possession of
My soul as a moveable thing.

Jennifer Hooper

Miss Story

Miss York Miss England
Minority winning Misses
Nobody expects you to be
A bohemian rhapsody in this:
women's hair-framed faces are a visual melody
in the ordinary understanding of races,
until news-reading talking heads of white stereotype
add a race-ripping like
the wind that blows,
a wind of change
over who is 'the Miss'?
Who will they help with this?
Black and mixed economies, charities or only generalities?
Should Miss have challenged Jagger's Brown Sugar
of ages ago? Because sugar sells itself now,
as if men don't exist!
Some points the young might miss?
Is hair and skin just ratio?
Curl to curl?
Iron to iron?
Surely it's offensive to mention
Coffee and Caramel?
A cultural gravy train that men will fight for their place on:
there's a timer on board identity so that others can benefit
and be born.
Relationships under wraps, until ratio has been agreed?
Ratio, nearly a creed?
Poker straight, poker face
Cat walk to human walk and back again,
Evolution has needs.
Camera to mirror
Roots to reality,
ratio will not do to describe what's me or you!
Maths, Science and human essence or

Statistics out for the lads?
Who creates winners, indirectly asks
about losers, choosers
What about history?
Is it all gone in a Miss Story?

Emma Louise Felicia Hopkins

Talking Peacock

How do you live?
Where do you live?
On my head
For my body
What must you be?
Hair and skin is all they see
But I made you sound like an insect
Leave out the 'in' and I might be quite right
A sect of hair and skin are the presence
of women, unless they have a fight
and might that needs a brain,
beyond the Peacock issues of hair and skin
should be background, ethnicity, heritage
stories and intimacy.
As pulse not shadow: suspicion,
to scorch a Peacock, search for shadows no!
Peacock and shadows must fight
Where do you live?
How do you live?
Is might!
Should we talk a lot about what we've got?
When skin and hair created becomes
more of an issue than self-stating talk
The presence of different Peacocks
In a family or other gathering
Makes "lights on", "lights off" a philosophy!
Self is gone
If hair and skin is all along
what gets the gong, but don't forget them
for that's where the breeze can breeze:
don't forget the features that may
be played by cancer keys
Don't go blonde with weaves go blue
Is hair the lengths that women will go to?

Purple, silver, gold, bronze – metal tones
For 'The Matrix' by minority women,
But hair and skin philosophy espoused
Not a blonde bow
The future is now.

Emma Louise Felicia Hopkins

Colour Canvas

I paddle in a tug boat
Between cultures
Wanting to wear –
Traditional clothing?

Swapping fear for fact
My skin became
The canvass
Of the ancestors

Why try to differentiate
Between Gaelic and Patois
I make no distinction

Fortune tellers and gypsies
Are drawn towards me
Feeling the intricacy of my soul

Palms crossed with silver
Bestow upon me
Rabbit feet, four leaved clover
Horse shoes, and bunches of heather

Witch doctors rattle shells
Sprinkle herbal powders
Chant a path around my feet

I am the meeting point
The crossing of cultures
The evidence of my forefathers

Each of my palms
Bare two life lines

Michelle Hubbard

Lost for Words

"You've been in the sun along time,"
he stated, followed
quickly with a chuckle
of embarrassment, or was it
real humour?

We sat, he looked and smiled at me; at my brown skin,
I looked back at him, at his dark skin
and in this moment, wished time, mad moments
were recordable, so as I could
rewind and delete.

Those words that way back then
I heard but had no words of my own
to voice back, to confront,
to challenge,
to defend

my black boyfriend,
the first time ever
for me to introduce
a real boyfriend,
this was serious

And yet he was
the one and only real
boyfriend that
I ever introduced
to my grandfather.

Nicole Moore

SKIN

Yours, mine, a tremendous outline
For creatures, for futures
For protection against the unknown
armour
against disclosing dreams

Skin, carries your spirit within
Skin acts as a barrier to whether I let you in
on
my portable journey
Adrift with its unnecessaries

Skin is a spectacular, flexible surface
Harmonious and bright
Reflecting past lives and perplexity
that slip
away when you aren't looking.

Nicole Moore

Back to Black

As a child I played
With my pearl faced doll
And imagined I was white
With blond hair
Tasting that uneasy longing
For the absence of pigment

A shared desire secretly held
By black and blackened sisters
Rarely admitted in white circles

In my teens I found out
I could never be white
So I settled for light
Instead became 'light skinned'
Colloquially 'red'
That said
I was beautied by it
Or so I thought
In the blinkered eyes
Of internalised
Racism

I fell in love with whiteness
In the form of a man
Thought happiness had found me
Or I it
But it was short-lived

For some ivory 'saint'
Very kindly opened his eyes
To my audacious genes
And their tendency to out-colour
Theirs

In any progeny
Of our unity

With that
He awoke from his dream
And ended our relationship
And so it was
That in the winter
Of my twenty-fifth year
I became black

Norma Treasure-Garwood

AUTHOR BIOGRAPHIES

Ellen Aaku
Ellen is a Zambian born in the UK. Her short stories have been published in anthologies in Australia, South Africa and the US. Her book *Wandi's Little Voice,* won the 2004 Macmillan's New Children's Writer Award. In 2007 her story *Sozi's Box* won the Commonwealth Short Story Competition.

Marcellina Aderibigbe
Marcellina was born in London to Nigerian parents. A Training Administrator by profession, who is still in the process of developing her writing and cultivating the craft. She draws inspiration from life around her. Writing enables Marcellina to initiate a lyrical conversation and to think things through.

Louisa Adjoa-Parker
Louisa is a poet and black history writer who runs *Adjoa Consultancy,* which aims to explore stories of diverse people through Literature, History and the Arts. Louisa's collection *Salt-sweat and Te*ars was published to critical acclaim by Cinnamon Press in 2007. Her poem 'Rag Doll' was highly commended by the Forward Prize 2008.

Gennett Aku Agbenu
Gennett was born in Berlin, Germany. She studied Graphic

Design at the Merz-Akademie in Stuttgart. Her final project concentrated on the medial representation of black hair and the influence of tradition, identity and politics on black hair-styles today. Since 2005 she has worked for several publishing houses, design and branding agencies in England and Germany.

Natalie Ambersley

Natalie grew up in London with her mum, dad and sister. Her main passion is writing, in particular Arts and Culture. In 2008 she worked at *Pride* magazine and now writes for a number of online publications. She is currently writing a novel based on her dad's life in Jamaica.

Catherine Anthony Boldeau

Catherine has an MA in Creative Writing. She is also a member of the Chartered Institute of Journalists and has written hundreds of published articles. She currently lectures in Creative Writing, Acting and Performance, Literacy and Music.

Patsy Antoine

Patsy is a writer, editor and literary consultant. She has had creative fiction and non-fiction published in *Best* magazine, *Sexual Attraction Revealed* and in the forthcoming *Tell Tales 4 – Global Village*. Her short story *Jah Goat Finds Liberty* was longlisted in the 2005 Bridport prize.

Margaret Auguste

A writer, therapist, librarian and mother of four, Margaret has engaged abused children in therapy, has encouraged a love of reading to her students and most importantly supported and nurtured her active family of four. Margaret has an MA in Psychology and has written for websites, literary and multicultural journals. She lives in New Jersey, US.

Scherin Barlow Massay

Scherin was born in Guyana, South America. She is a

researcher, writer and visual artist and has had several poems published.

Daniella Blechner
Daniella is a London based Writer/Director whose real writing journey began by writing comedy sketches for Youth Project *Phenomenon '98* featuring Gina Yashere and Richard Blackwood. She then graduated from Ravensbourne College in 2004 where she wrote, produced and directed her first short *Connexions,* which was Nominated for Best Screenplay at the BFM Short Film Awards in 2006.

Nehanda Buchanan
Nehanda is a mother of three; born in Clapham, grew up in Croydon, now residing in North London. Nehanda's work experience has been mainly in Education providing Careers Guidance. Her first published article was printed in November 2006 News check issue entitled *In Pursuit of Happiness* 30 interviews on fulfilling careers.

Monique Campbell
Monique is a London-born writer. Her work has appeared in *Decode Magazine*, anthologies such as *Brown Eyes* and *Sexual Attraction Revealed*. Monique has articles published on websites including *www.literatenubian.org* and *www.fiba-filmbank.org*

Christine Collymore
Christine was born in England, of Caribbean descent and is a single parent in her forties, residing in Northamptonshire. Her love of writing began twenty years ago. But only recently has she considered allowing the wider public to see her work. 'I hope the piece(s) in this anthology arouse thinking, questioning and emotions.'

Leaya Collymore
Leaya is 13. From the age of 11, Leaya found that poetry let her

imagination wander and be free. One of Leaya's interests is music. She enjoys all types but mostly prefers soca. Leaya plays various instruments and currently is learning to play the tuba.

Dorothy Cornibert du Boulay

The poem *Jan Blan Hair* was inspired by the life and work of Langston Hughes. Previous writing includes the screenplay *War Inna Babylon* and the essay *Searching for a Black Jesus*. Dorothy is currently working on a documentary about inter war Black British insurgency and Pan Africanism.

Suzanne Creaville

Suzanne has written fiction pieces and poems with a biographical and cultural slant. Her short autobiography *Afro Child* has been adapted over the years to reflect the changing nature of contemporary life and perspective. Suzanne is of Guyanese descent and lives in South East London.

Yolande Deane

Yolande is 34 and from Tottenham in north London. Her parents come from the Caribbean. Yolande is an EFL (English as a Foreign Language) teacher. Other than writing during her free time she fences and practices Tai Chi on a regular basis.

Tjawangwa Dema

Tjawangwa is a Botswana based writer, performance poet and workshop facilitator. She is a 2005/06 British Council Crossing Borders participant, 2007/08 Power in the Voice mentor as well as a 2009 participant in the Cambridge Seminar on Contemporary Literature who has performed in Botswana, South Africa and India.

Chris-Tia Donaldson

Chris-Tia is the author of *Thank God I'm Natural: The Ultimate Guide to Caring for and Maintaining Natural Hair*. She has been featured in *USA Today*, the *Chicago Tribune*, the *Chicago Sun*

Times, and the *Detroit News*, for her thoughts on the growing natural hair trend, in addition to issues related to black women and their beauty spending habits.

Amanda Epe
Born and raised in north London, Amanda is a British-African. Amanda has worked as a British Airways cabin crew member, teacher and now works towards a career as a writer. This anthology opportunity has inspired her to take the WRITE stride to become the published writer of awaited manuscripts.

Karron Francis-Darling
Karron was born in England in 1963. Her parents sent her to Jamaica to live with her grandparents; she grew up in Kingston. At the age of 16, Karron migrated to New York where she completed her education and worked, returning to England in 1990. She now lives in London.

Leandra Gebrakedan
Leandra is the eldest of five children. She was born in Africa and raised in the UK from the age of five years old. Leandra worked previously in education and now wants to start her own business or write a book.

Donna-Marie Glashen
Donna-Marie has presented an academic essay on diversity for the European Union in Berlin. Her play, *Illusions of Grandeur* was broadcast on Radio 5 and her articles have been published in *New Nations* Newspaper, *BFM* and *Calabash Literary Magazine*. She is co-founder of *Living Fruits*, a collective of emerging female writers.

Nicola Greenwood
Nicola is a Bristol born London dweller who began writing as a child on everything from the wallpaper behind a wardrobe to napkins at dinner, revealing the carvings of her perception in

poetry. Her love of language, filled with the beauty, expression, clarity and confusion of words, continues to grow.

Zakia Henderson-Brown

Born and raised in Brooklyn, New York, Zakia is a poet and community organizer. She is a fellow of the North Country Institute for Writers of Color; recipient of a full-tuition residency scholarship at the Fine Arts Work Center in Provincetown, MA; and has works forthcoming in *Torch*. She hopes to inspire and enact transformation through her poems and social justice work.

Tracy Henry

Tracy is a natural black woman, London born and raised, descended from Dominica. Tracy writes songs of different genres and fictional poetry about real issues. Tracy's work *Nothing new* has been published in the *Voice* newspaper's Poet's corner. Tracy has a catalogue of songs and poems ready and waiting to be published.

Louise Hercules

Louise is a London based artist who specialises in both poetry and photography. Louise's dynamic body of work explores provocative themes such as: identity, gender and relationships through the use of sensual imagery and dramatic dialogue which permeate throughout her artwork.

Jennifer Hooper

Jennifer was born in 1964; culture Black British, raised in West London. Her writing interests are autobiographical poetry fused with psychotherapy. Her writing is a form that focuses on aspects of relationships, love, hate, loss, pain and conflict to find meaning. Poetry is her art form for processing her fantasies.

Emma Louise Felicia Hopkins

Two mixed race parents of West African and Lebanese ethnicity provide Emma with an epic sense of identity and writing, which includes enough poetry for a collection, short stories and pseudonyms NOTTA VIKING and Amy G. Dala (via amygdala brain function) supports her Machiavellian sensibility.

Michelle 'The Mother' Hubbard

Michelle is a poet/workshop facilitator, passionate about poetry, regularly appearing around the UK, reciting her poetry on radio, and delivering creative workshops. She is a Founder member of Nottingham's Blackdrop open mic. Michelle has successfully self published *The Tapestry of a Black Woman* & *The Irish-Jamaican*, and has won several poetry competitions and 'Slams'.

Rachelle Hull

Born and raised in London, of Jamaican parentage, Rachelle is a writer and freelance journalist, who is passionate about film, literature and yogurt coated pretzels. She is currently working on a collection of short-story fiction, exploring the joys and oddities of relationships.

Anduosjahla James-Wheatle

Anduosjahla completed a BA Hons in Social Policy and Sociology at Royal Holloway, University of London. Anduosjahla's career involves supporting young people and their families. She has written poetry, theatrical scripts and directed theatrical productions. Anduosjahla enjoys the arts, and is currently rekindling a relationship with writing again....

Fiona Joseph

Fiona is a former lecturer and textbook author now running an online educational publishing company. Since joining the National Academy of Writing (NAW) in 2008 she has had two stories published in anthologies and was recently awarded the *NAW 2009 Prize for Fiction*. She blogs for emerging writers at: *www.fionajoseph.com*

Colette Machado is a journalist, wife and mother of two young boys. She currently works as an online news journalist for BBC

News Online (London), and regularly writes features and news articles for various publications and websites. She has ten years experience of teaching a beginners' journalism course to young people in east London.

Dr Sheree Mack
Sheree successfully completed her PhD in Creative Writing at Newcastle University in December 2009. She is an active freelance writer within the UK, having worked with, among others, *Creative Partnerships Durham Sunderland, Cumbria and Northumberland, Arts UK, Diamond Twig, Durham Literature Festival, Apples and Snakes, Malika's Kitchen* and *New Writing North.*

Dr Valerie Mason-John
Valerie is the author of the award winning novel – *The Banana Kid*, named as the British Color Purple. She is also author of the self help book *Detox Your Heart*, working with anger, fear and hatred. She is currently working on the adaptation of her novel to screen, and her second novel *Destinations. www.valeriemason-john.co.uk*

Fiona Mckinson
Fiona is a creative writer and published freelance journalist based in South London. She has an MA in Journalism Studies. Her poetry was previously published in the first two *Shangwe* anthologies as well as *The Voice* newspaper and the *New Nation Newspaper. www.thetalentshow.co.uk*

Mesha Mcneil
Mesha Mcneil is a young writer who is just starting out in the field. Mesha is currently studying for a degree in English Literature at the University of East Anglia where she will graduate in July 2010. She is an intern for Words of Colour Productions, where she is gaining invaluable journalistic experience.

Nicole Moore
Nicole is of Guyanese and English parentage. She is a writer/editor

and published poet, with experience of producing work for magazines and poetry anthologies. She is the editor of *Brown Eyes* (2005) and *Sexual Attraction Revealed* (2007) both Shangwe produced anthologies of creative expressions by black & mixed-race women. Nicole is a member of The Society of Authors. She lives in north London.

Bola Odeyemi

Bola holds a BA in Broadcast Journalism and an MA in Communications, Culture and Society from Nottingham Trent University and Goldsmiths College respectively. She currently works as a Communications Officer for a NGO which focuses on education in Africa. She started writing poetry in 2005 as a hobby and for creative expression.

Cristina Odigie-Bulnes

Born in England to a black Nigerian father and a white Spanish mother, Cristina grew up in Spain where her family relocated. With a business and financial background, she's training as an Integrative Child Psychotherapist in London. Writing since a young age, she's inspired by art and travel.

Elayne Ogbeta

Ever since Elayne was ten, she knew she wanted to be a writer. Elayne lives in Salford with two bubbly children and a supportive hubby. She also teaches 16-18 year olds. Elayne wants to dedicate *Rapunzel, Rapunzel*, to all those black women who appreciate the versatility of their hair!

Akuba Quansah

Awarding-winning Ghanaian artiste, Akuba, was born in 1960s London. Having lectured in several academic institutions since 1988, she currently facilitates storytelling workshops for the British Museum. She has written numerous folktales, rhymes, poems and has contributed to eight anthologies including American publication, *Journeys Home* (2009). Supported by the

Positive Awareness Charity and Ealing Council she founded a **W**riting, **A**cting and **P**ublishing **P**roject for **Y**oungsters.

Dorothea Smart

Dorothea's most recent poetry collection *Ship Shape* (Peepal Tree, 2008), is considered "among the best of her generation". In 2009, as an African Writers Abroad [PEN] member, she was commissioned to write on climate change and justice and was a guest at the Badilisha Poetry Xchange, Cape Town.

Norma Treasure-Garwood

Norma is a former local radio presenter and black theatre marketeer. She ran a Marketing Consultancy for several years in Birmingham. While chief executive of a successful black mentoring programme she helped to pioneer mentoring for black students/employees in the UK. Norma writes poetry in her spare time.

Pauline Walker

Pauline is black-British, born and brought up in the UK. She has recently taken up creative writing. Pauline is currently writing her first novel and is also working on a screenplay for a short film.

Brenda White

Brenda's interest in drama and performing has taken her in many directions since studying a B-Tec National Diploma in Performing Arts in 1994. Her career experiences range from acting roles, coordinating events, to working with young people, and directing plays for the stage. Brenda enjoys creating new ideas, using drama or literature.

Yvonne Witter

Yvonne is a self employed Business Consultant specialising in helping people start and grow their own business. Success as a parent, is her greatest achievement apart from surviving the vagaries of life; life as a journey. Her favourite quote: 'there is no power without responsibility'.

ACKNOWLEDGMENTS

I would like to thank the hair stories blog contributors who participated in a Black History Month project 2008 and provided evidence that the subject of our hair was definitely worth writing about.

Many thanks to the Arts Council England, London, for the financial support and to David Cross, Literary Officer, who helped me enhance my proposal by discussing the project. Receiving the funding to fulfil this endeavour is a sign that the themes of hair and skin are being taken seriously and that our voices will be heard.

One important lesson learned throughout my professional and personal life is the importance of gratitude – there have been many supportive conversations sometimes with complete strangers, who have patted me on the back when they found out what I was working on.

Thanks must go to the volunteer support received from Sheree Mack and Patsy Antoine who ensured supportive dialogue and mutual artistic development took place so that the project achieved high-quality work throughout. I would particularly like to thank Aisha Badmus who volunteered her time copy editing some of the personal essays.

Many thanks to all the contributors of this anthology that I feel honoured and privileged to have made contact with – a few good friends have come out of this too!

To my writing buddy Christine Collymore – thank you for our fortnightly telephone 'meetings', which sometimes became quite heated.

I cannot leave out my son Andrew Moore, who has been there in the background and foreground discussing book titles, helping take photos, etc. Thank you.

Last but not least, I would like to thank Akuba Quansah, who is a great friend with mutual interests and a true fan of Shangwe – who has consistently shared her insights into the project's development.